The Endangered Environment

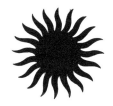

Compiled by
ASHLEY MONTAGU

Mason & Lipscomb PUBLISHERS NEW YORK

To the Memory of
Zabelle Sourian

Library of Congress Cataloging in Publication Data

Montagu, Ashley, 1905-   comp.
   The endangered environment.

   Bibliography: p.
   1. Environmental health. I. Title.
RA565.M66 1974   614.7   74-4180
ISBN 0-88405-027-0

Contents

Epigraph

... The devastation of the environment is at bottom a result of the kind of society we have built and the kind of people we are. ... To arrest the deterioration of the environment it will be necessary to control many of the same forces which have prevented us from ending the war in Indochina or giving justice to black Americans. ...

... [Most] of the talk about the environmental crisis that turns on the word *pollution,* as if we face a cosmic-scale problem of sanitation, is grossly misleading. What confronts us is an extreme imbalance between society's hunger—the rapidly growing sum of human wants —and the limited capacities of the earth.

—Leo Marx, "American Institutions and Ecological Ideals," *Science,* Vol. 170, No. 3961 (November 27, 1970), pp. 951, 952.

Consider, for example, the fate of prime agricultural lands on the borders of our burgeoning cities. What happens when a landowner is offered a small fortune by a developer? What agency protects the public interest from the irretrievable loss of topsoil that requires centuries to produce? Who sees to it that housing, factories, highways, and shopping centers are situated on the far more plentiful sites where nothing edible will ever grow? The answer is that no such agencies exist, and the market principle is allowed to rule. Since World War II approximately one-fifth of California's invaluable farm land has been lost in this way. Here, as in many cases of air and water pollution, the dominant motive of our business system—private profit—leads to the violation of ecological standards.

—Marx, "American Institutions and Ecological Ideals," *Science* (November 27, 1970), p. 948.

1

Introduction

As a result of man's activities, the environment is in danger of total destruction.

This may sound like an extreme statement. Unfortunately, it is not. Great bodies of water—Lake Erie for instance—have already been literally destroyed; others, such as lakes Michigan and Superior, are threatened. Rivers that flow in the vicinity of most cities are so polluted it would take centuries and vast sums of money to restore them to something resembling their natural state. The cities themselves have been so abused they have become virtually unmanageable, ungovernable, and unlivable. In our large cities not only is the air unsafe but it is no longer safe to walk at night, and in some places not even in broad daylight. Compared to our urban areas, the jungle is in every way a far safer and a much healthier place.

Almost everywhere the air is polluted with the poisonous gases emanating from automobiles, from the stacks of industrial plants, and from the burning of refuse. And what refuse cannot be incinerated is taken out to sea and dumped there, where it pollutes the coastal waters, destroys oyster beds, and injures fisheries. Tankers carrying the oil that eventually produces much of the pollution of the air on land leak their lethal cargo into the sea. And shipwrecks involving such vessels spew millions of gallons of oil into the sea and onto beaches, killing or injuring every living thing it touches.

Meanwhile, the oil barons, with their government oil-depletion allowances, resist every attempt to develop a nongasoline-burning engine; our roadbuilders, with the encouragement of the government in the form of huge subsidies, go merrily on destroying the countryside, laying waste the land, so that the millions of motor vehicles may more pervasively and effectively continue to add to the pollution and destruction of the land.

Perhaps the single most disastrous invention of man has proven to be the internal combustion engine—as the following pages of this book make so abundantly clear. Altogether, apart from its damaging environmental effects, the internal-combustion-engined vehicle has served to bring about more destructive social changes than any other invention of the last 500 years. It has virtually destroyed the extended family, it has atomized and sequestrated the nuclear family, it has largely served to remove the father from the family, it has scattered members of the extended family far and wide so that communication between them has been reduced to a minimum, human relations have become as flat and arid and dehumanized as the roads upon which the motor vehicles rush madly by.

Millions drive to and from work along freeways often so thickly congested with traffic that "insanity" becomes the only proper word with which to describe the trauma—man no longer capable of governing his own affairs. Helicopters, adding both to the congestion and pollution in the skies above, broadcast the traffic conditions on the roads and bridges below, while the drivers on the congested roads sit behind their wheels fuming and fretting, suffering the strains and stresses of frustration that will exacerbate the psychosomatic disorders that constitute the occupational hazard of contemporary living and working in the city. Breathing the poisoned air, they eventually reach their destinations, although in the course of so doing they further contribute to the load of toxins in the air. The presence of so many poison-producing vehicles, in addition to the destructive smog they produce, in many other ways adds to the stresses and strains of a madhouse already burdened with problems that grow worse every day.

No sane person, one would think, would continue to subject himself to such harassment, and no civilized person would continue to either work or live in such a place. Yet millions do, and most of them do so, to put it plainly, because they are trapped. Most people simply cannot get up and leave. In any event, where would they go? There are very few places left on this earth that have not been affected by technologized man. There are some pretty villages still left here and there, but most of them can scarcely manage to give employment even to their native-born inhabitants. Nor have such refuge areas managed to escape the automobile and its noxious exhalations.

The Isles of Illusion syndrome—that there exists somewhere on this earth a lovely island, free of all the curses of modern civilization, quiet, peaceful, green and tranquil—is indeed an illusion. Such places once did exist—the Hawaiian Islands, for example. But one now has only to visit Honolulu to see what a disaster civilized man has made of what at one time must have been very near paradise; the United States Army owns most of the land, and what it hasn't destroyed, the businessmen are rapidly turning into another Miami Beach. It is a very depressing experience.

Civilized man's effects upon the environment have everywhere been disastrous. If we ask why, the answer is simple: greed. Greed has been the universal driving force that has caused man to ravish the land. It is greed that is responsible for the environmental disasters created by technologized man. What did the great industrialists who for decades poured their poisonous refuse into Lake Erie care about the consequences to the lake? Their only care was profit. At the appropriate ceremonial occasions they would, of course, with deep-felt patriotic fervor, join in singing "America the Beautiful," but then that cost no money and little effort, and was strictly a matter of ritual incantation.

The biggest polluters and murderers of the environment always fly the flag from the highest mast, and to a man they are the most perfervid of patriots. But let us not be deceived. It is the big industrialists, the large corporations, the developers and exploiters, who are and have been the most serious offenders.

The average citizen, however, must bear his share of responsibility for the uncontrolled degradation of the environment, if only because of his complacency and compliance. The citizen has it within his power to stop the rapine and destruction of the land. He has the vote and he has the power to organize the voices and the power of likeminded citizens to bring the proper pressure to bear upon the legislators of his State and of his nation. It is the obligation of the responsible citizen to be informed and to act, and not to fall back as so many do upon a handwashing indifference which leaves the necessary action to the other fellow.

Freedom is the right to be able to do what you ought, and in no land does the citizen enjoy that freedom more than in America. This is a fact that all of us had better come to understand and do something about before it is too late. The earth, given to us as a trust to keep healthy and green, is a trust we have abused. We must stop the abusers from continuing in their lethal activities, for unless they are stopped the earth will die. Detailed controls must be instituted for everyone relating to the use of the environment, from littering the sidewalks to every other form of possible environmental abuse. These controls must have the force of law and the power of government behind them.

It is far better to institute laws and regulations designed to prevent the abuse of the environment rather than introduce laws that simply control the abuse. In short, pollutant-free fuels should be developed so that polluting fuels can be abolished as completely as possible. No one should be permitted to be in a position to empty any kind of deleterious matter into any body of water or air. There have been laws on the books for many years designed to prevent the pollution of water and air, but no one has been concerned enough until recently to see that they were enforced. So, clearly, laws are not enough. Laws are necessary, but they are not sufficient conditions for an effective program of prevention and control. The involved citizen is the most essential of the necessary conditions. To help the ordinary citizen (and we are all ordinary citizens) become aware of the seriousness of the problem and its urgency, I have compiled the data relating to the various aspects of environmental damage, in the hope that the reader armed with the necessary information will be stimulated to do what he can toward preventing the further deterioration of the environment. This is the principal purpose of this book.

The data presented in the pages which follow has been deliberately maintained in the form which keeps each statement of the facts as short and as clear as possible. Such succinctness lends itself to both easy remembering and ready quotability. The source of each statement is cited briefly at the end of each quotation and full bibliographic information is given at the end of the book. It is hoped that this book will serve as a convenient source-book for writers, speakers, publicists, and all others who care about the quality of the world in which they and their children are to live. It is my hope, also, that the book may find a wide readership in our schools and colleges.

To Dr. Philip Gordon I owe thanks for his kindness in reading the proofs.

Ashley Montagu

Princeton, New Jersey

2

Air Pollution

＊

The average person breathes 35 pounds of air each day—6 times as much as the food and drink he consumes.

—*Needed: Clean Air*, U.S. Department of Health, Education, and Welfare (Washington, D.C., 1969), Publication No. 138–E–5–69, p. 3.

In the United States we pollute our air with "aerial garbage."

—*Needed: Clean Air*, p. 4.

Toxic matter is being released into the air at a rate of about 200 million tons a year, or nearly a ton for every American.

—*Environmental Health Problems*, U.S. Public Health Service, U.S. Department of Health, Education, and Welfare (Washington, D.C., 1970), Publication No. 0–380–961, p. 4.

Though containing pollutants, the cleanest air on earth occurs over the middle of the ocean. In contrast with this, rural air has 10 times more pollution; the air over small towns, 35 times more; and the air over cities, 150 times more.

—Howard R. Lewis, *With Every Breath You Take* (New York: Crown, 1965), pp. 4–5.

While few Americans realize it, we are experiencing a worsening shortage of clean air. The amount of air actually available to a community is often limited by weather and terrain. Thus, we human beings are competing with sources of pollution for the use of a restricted air supply.

So far, the pollutants are winning. Even beyond the flood of customary wastes—from cars, furnaces, industry—complex chemical compounds are being introduced into industrial processes at an increasing rate each year. Most such compounds find their way into the air —and into your lungs. Their poisonous properties may be learned only after serious damage occurs.

—Lewis, *With Every Breath You Take*, p. xvi.

Each one of us needs about 480 cubic feet of fresh air each 24 hours. . . . Unfortunately, however, the combined forces of our technological society and our general carelessness have launched a massive assault on fresh air so that, according to the National Air Pollution Control Administration, there isn't any uncontaminated air left in this country.

—Betty Ann Ottinger, *What Every Woman Should Know—and do—About Pollution: A Guide to Good Global Housekeeping* (Washington, D.C.: EP Press, 1970), p. 20.

Every day, a major diversified industrial center, as defined by the Public Health Service, can expect to be deluged by at least 574 tons of pollutants from these industrial sources: From ceramics industries, 11 tons of dust and 2 tons of gas; from iron and steel production, 22 tons of dust and 2 tons of gas; from iron and steel processing, 12 tons of dust and 2 tons of gas; from noniron metal processing, 5 tons of dust and 97 tons of gas; from the production and processing of plastics and chemicals, 63 tons of dust and 162 tons of gas; from food processing, 3 tons of dust and 27 tons of gas; from paint manufacturing, 2 tons of dust and 137 tons of gas; and from the production and processing of concrete products and paving materials, 26 tons of dust and 1 ton of gas.

—Lewis, *With Every Breath You Take*, p. 43.

In Chicago alone, the total emission of pollutants [into the air] is estimated at 25,000 tons a day; in Los Angeles, at 8,600 tons a day; in Greater Detroit, at 4,920 tons a day; in metropolitan Buffalo, New York, at 2,740 tons a day; in Portland, Oregon, at 873 tons a day.

—Lewis, *With Every Breath You Take*, p. 43.

10

In all, some degree of chemical fallout in the United States afflicts an estimated 7,273 communities, where live at least 107,600,000 people—some 60 percent of the nation's population.

The United States Public Health Service estimates that no less than 43 million people (some 24 percent of all Americans) live in communities having major air pollution problems. Altogether this takes in 308 cities with populations of 2,500 or more. It includes all five cities (New York, Chicago, Los Angeles, Philadelphia, and Detroit) with populations of 1,000,000 or more; 11 of the 16 cities with populations between 500,000 and 1,000,000; and 13 of the 30 cities with populations between 250,000 and 500,000.

In addition, some 30 million other people live in 850 other cities with air contamination that is somewhat less severe but too serious to be classified as minor.

—Lewis, *With Every Breath You Take*, p. 2.

Air pollutants may occur in the form of gases, liquids, and solids, both singly and in combination. Gaseous pollutants make up about 90 percent of the total mass emitted to the atmosphere with particulates and aerosols accounting for the remaining 10 percent. Small particulates are of particular importance because they may be in the respirable size range. These small particles may contain biologically active elements and compounds. Furthermore, they tend to remain in the atmosphere where they interfere with both solar and terrestrial infrared radiation, which may affect climate on a global basis.

—George B. Morgan, Guntis Ozolins, and Elbert C. Tabor, "Air Pollution Surveillance Systems," *Science*, Vol. 170, No. 3955 (October 16, 1970), pp. 295–96.

. . . [Among] the rather universal effects of [air] pollutants on local climates . . . is the attenuation of solar radiation by suspended particulates. Although this affects the whole spectrum, it is most pronounced in the short wavelengths. The total direct radiation over most major cities is weakened by about 15 percent, sometimes more in winter and less in summer. The ultraviolet light is reduced by 30 percent, on an average, and in winter often no radiation of wavelengths below 390 nanometers is received.

—Helmut E. Landsberg, "Man-Made Climatic Changes," *Science*, Vol. 170, No. 3964 (December 18, 1970), p. 1271.

11

Horizontally, the particulate haze [in polluted air] interferes with visibility in cities. When shallow temperature inversions are present, the accumulation of aerosols can cause 80- or 90-percent reduction of the visual range as compared with the range for the general uncontaminated environment.

—Landsberg, "Man-Made Climatic Changes," *Science* (December 18, 1970), p. 1272.

. . . [The eastern seaboard] megalopolis is often so thickly overcast with pollutants that no portion of its 645-mile length can be navigated visually from the air. What disturbs health authorities is not so much that airline pilots cannot see through that [pollutant] soup but that the people down below are breathing it.

—Lewis, *With Every Breath You Take*, p. 5.

. . . [There] are but five basic types of air pollution. These types are characterized by the emission [into the air] of (1) odor, (2) dust, (3) smoke, (4) motor exhaust, or (5) toxic substances. Most instances of air pollution contain more than one of these characteristics.

—Lewis, *With Every Breath You Take*, p. 44.

Dr. Robert M. Senior, Director, Pulmonary Division, Department of Medicine, the Jewish Hospital of St. Louis, and Assistant Professor of Medicine, Washington University School of Medicine: . . . The major pollutants [of the atmosphere] recognized now are carbon monoxide, sulfur oxides, hydrocarbons, nitrogen oxides, and particulate matter. In our environment the primary sources of air pollution are (1) automobiles, (2) space heating, (3) power utilities, (4) industrial processing and manufacturing, and (5) refuse disposal. The automobile is by far the single most important hazard and is responsible for most of the pollution from carbon monoxide, hydrocarbons, and nitrogen oxides.

—"The Role of Air Pollution in Chronic Obstructive Pulmonary Disease," *Journal of the American Medical Association* (hereafter *JAMA*), Vol. 214, No. 5 (November 2, 1970), pp. 894–95.

Upward of 100 specific substances have been identified as pollutants; many other pollutants have been detected, but not analyzed and identified. Among the known pollutants are at least 20 metallic elements. Most are damaging to health. Other pollutants are organic compounds. These contain a nearly infinite number of combinations of carbon with hydrogen and other elements. Among organic pollutants are some that cause cancer.

—Lewis, *With Every Breath You Take*, p. 39.

Gases and particulates may undergo a variety of reactions to produce secondary pollutants that in some cases are more toxic than the parent pollutants. This is particularly true in the case of photochemical smog.

—Morgan, Ozolins, and Tabor, "Air Pollution Surveillance Systems," *Science* (October 16, 1970), p. 296.

Pollutant concentrations [in the air] are directly related to the density of industry and the use of fossil fuels for power and space heating. Cities that have poor ventilation or frequent temperature inversions are most plagued by air pollution episodes.

—Morgan, Ozolins, and Tabor, "Air Pollution Surveillance Systems," *Science* (October 16, 1970), p. 296.

. . . [The] amount of air available to a given community at a given time is not infinite but rather may be severely restricted by local weather and terrain. . . .

If all cities were situated at the tops of hills, and if the wind always blew, air pollution at worst would be merely a minor nuisance. But such is not the condition, and few communities are lucky enough to have adequate ventilation. . . .

. . . [The] atmosphere is extremely shallow compared to the bulk of the earth. . . . The inhabitable portion of the atmosphere, which alone contains fully half the molecules in the air, would compare to the earth like the skin of an apple. . . .

. . . In practical terms, it makes little difference what the general quantity of air is. What does count is how much is available to a given locale compared with how much is required by the human beings on one hand and by sources of air pollution on the other.

—Lewis, *With Every Breath You Take,* pp. 22–24.

The city system from Richmond, Virginia, to Portland, Maine, . . . is generally an area of weak winds. . . . This means, concludes Dr. Landsberg [Helmut E. Landsberg, director of the U.S. Weather Bureau's Office of Climatology], that pollutants will stay concentrated in the general district of which these cities are centers. Within the 645-mile strip live 38 million people . . . who thus must breathe perhaps the most densely, continuously and extensively polluted air in the world.

—Lewis, *With Every Breath You Take,* p. 29.

The air available for use by a community may be further limited by a thermal inversion, a weather phenomenon that often accompanies an interval of windlessness. . . .

. . . In one form of inversion, the air stays at the same temperature —or even becomes progressively warmer—for considerable distances from ground level up. In such cases there are no upward air currents —and pollutants collect near the ground. In another form of inversion, the air becomes cooler, as would be normal. But, not far up [in the atmosphere], a layer of warm air intervenes. This inversion layer obstructs the upward air currents. Pollutants then strike a low ceiling and accumulate in the now limited air space underneath. . . .

An inversion, in combination with general windlessness, has been a factor of all air pollution disasters.

—Lewis, *With Every Breath You Take,* pp. 30–31.

. . . [One] especially troublesome feature of inversions caused by high-pressure systems . . . [is that] they usually occur in cool, if not freezing, weather. Thus, when conditions are least satisfactory for dispersing pollutants, the burning of fuels for heat pours extra quantities of contaminants into the air.

—Lewis, *With Every Breath You Take,* pp. 32–33.

Once an inversion begins, the only way to alleviate the emergency (it cannot be stopped, except by a change in the weather) is for an entire city literally to shut down—heating units and electrical generators burning coal and oil have to go off—and all forms of combustion must cease. Automobiles must come to a dead halt. The dilemma, of course, is this: which will kill or injure more people, the air pollution emergency or the termination of essential services?

What all this means is that there is no such thing as "planning" for the [air pollution] emergency. . . .

—John C. Esposito, *Vanishing Air* (New York: Grossman, 1970), p. 5.

. . . [In] many American cities, a particularly bad combination of circumstances might, in any year, bring people to clutching at their throats and falling on the floor. Such cities have cut their margin of safety too fine. In a sense, what we should really have, is what we actually may have—a spectacular disaster. If a thousand people died in the street in one afternoon, and ten thousand were hauled off to be laid in hospital corridors, real action would result. Those who died would be martyrs. As it now goes, many millions of people may be dragging along at a reduced level of activity, failing to get the most out of their lives, because the American dream has vanished somewhere behind a yellowish, ill-smelling haze.

—George R. Stewart, *Not as Rich as You Think* (Boston: Houghton Mifflin, 1967), pp. 185–86.

Airline pilots report regularly sighting an envelope of pollution, ranging from 2,000 to 30,000 feet in depth, covering much of the United States.

—Lewis, *With Every Breath You Take*, p. 36.

In late October of 1963, a stagnant air mass over the northeastern United States caused a steady increase in pollution levels from Richmond, Virginia, to Boston. Though weather conditions were similar to those that caused the London smog that killed 4,000 persons, the buildup in the United states covered an enormously greater area.

For several days levels of toxic gases in the air of New York and Philadelphia were more than five times normal. If we had not been lucky, and if this mass of contaminated air had not been blown out over the ocean, an incredibly large segment of our population might have died. Only the caprice of a wind saved us from a disaster.

—Lewis, *With Every Breath You Take*, p. xvii.

So great is the burden of pollution that were it not for the prevailing wind, New York City might have gone the way of Sodom and Gomorrah. As [noted in] a 1966 report to Mayor Lindsay [*Freedom to Breathe, The Mayor's Task Force Report on Air Pollution*], "These [prevailing] winds are all that have spared the City an unspeakable tragedy. If New York had the sheltered topography of Los Angeles, everyone in this city would long since have perished from the poisons in the air." Occasionally the prevailing winds fail, a thermal inversion falls upon the city and 8 million New Yorkers find themselves trapped under a blanket of lethal smog. The first such episode recorded in New York City occurred in 1953 and took two to three hundred lives. . . . [It] was followed by similar, if less severe, occurrences in 1962, 1963, and 1966.

—Esposito, *Vanishing Air*, pp. 204–205.

Winds in the [Los Angeles] Basin are extremely weak, averaging only 6.2 miles per hour. For about 270 days a year, cooler air flows down the mountains, floating an inversion across the Basin like an airtight cover. . . . The inversion sometimes hangs so low that all pollutants are trapped in an airspace a mere 30 feet high.

—Lewis, *With Every Breath You Take*, p. 33.

Through the late fall of 1969 and the winter of 1969–70, Chicago experienced three, four, or maybe five air pollution episodes.

The actual number is uncertain, according to Chicago's . . . Director [of the Department of Air Pollution Control], Wallace M. Poston. Notwithstanding the Telemetered Air Monitoring Network (with third-generation computers), Poston . . . [said] that he was not sure how to define an episode.

—Esposito, *Vanishing Air*, p. 7.

State and city officials in New York City have defined air pollution emergencies out of existence.

On October 31, 1968, Mayor John V. Lindsay signed an executive order establishing a four-stage "Air Pollution Control Alert Warning System." The first stage, known as "Forecast," is merely a get-ready signal and is triggered by a Weather Bureau advisory that a high air pollution potential will exist for the next thirty-six hours. The following stages, called "Alert," "Warning," and "Emergency" are triggered as the concentrations of carbon monoxide, sulfur dioxide, and fine particulate matter reach designated levels. The triggering levels for the Emergency stage are set so high that one can say with almost total certainty that New York City will never again experience an air pollution emergency—at least it won't be called by that name. . . .

Before any automobile is banned from the streets, before any factory is completely shut down, and before all garbage incineration is brought to a halt, a condition of Emergency must be declared. The Emergency stage is reached only after average SO_2 [sulfur dioxide] levels equal or exceed .625 ppm [parts per million] for a twenty-four-hour period. By that definition, the famous New York City Thanksgiving Day episode of 1966, which snuffed out 150 to 175 lives, would not qualify as an emergency.

—Esposito, *Vanishing Air*, pp. 205–6.

Trouble [from severe air pollution] may well loom for Los Angeles, which sits in a smoggy bowl that often contains only 300 ft. of air. Almost every other day, the city's public schools forbid children to exercise lest they breathe too deeply.

—"Fighting to Save the Earth from Man," *Time* (February 2, 1970), p. 59.

As a word, *smog* was coined in the twentieth century, being an obvious blend of *smoke* and *fog*. The word has had a triumphant career. The chief trouble with it is that its suggestion has proved to be wholly inaccurate. As a great amount of highly technical research has demonstrated, fog has really nothing to do with the case, and smoke, as such, very little. . . .

. . . [One] might state briefly that smog is a fog-like, haze-like stuff, with a characteristic yellow undertone, that gets into the air so thickly

17

as even to cut visibility. It makes your eyes run and irritates your respiratory passages. . . .

. . . [Smog] consists of certain gases, . . . chiefly carbon monoxide, the oxides of sulfur and of nitrogen, and certain of the hydrocarbons. In addition to the man-produced basic components, certain other compounds are formed from them in the air itself under the influence of sunlight. The most important of these is that three-atomed molecule of oxygen known as ozone. . . .

. . . [There] are other components, such as fluorides and ketene. . . .

—Stewart, *Not as Rich as You Think,* pp. 179–82.

Ozone, a principal component of photochemical smog, discolors and disintegrates clothing and causes rubber to become brittle and crack. . . .

. . . Ozone and PAN [peroxyacyl nitrate] produce the eye irritation, coughing and chest soreness experienced by many Los Angeles residents on smoggy days.

—"Menace in the Skies," *Time* (January 27, 1967), p. 50.

. . . [The] experts are in fair agreement as to what is causing . . . [it]. First, there is transportation, that is, its almost universal motive power, the internal-combustion engine. Second, there are factories of many kinds and plants for generating electricity, together with the considerably less important heating plants and garbage-incinerators. . . .

. . . Transportation supplies nearly all the carbon monoxide (more than 90 percent of it), two-thirds of the hydrocarbons, and something more than one-third of the oxides of nitrogen. . . . Industry [all the non-transportation causes] . . . supplies . . . nearly all the oxides of sulfur, a third of the hydrocarbons, and two-thirds of the oxides of nitrogen.

—Stewart, *Not as Rich as You Think,* pp. 182–83.

Smog disintegrates nylon stockings in Chicago and Los Angeles, eats away historic stone statues and buildings in Venice and Cologne. Rapidly industrializing Denver, which for many years boasted of its crystalline air, is now often smogbound. In Whiting, Ind., a concentration of fog and pollution from an oil refinery produced a chemical mist that one night last year [1966] stripped paint from houses, turned others rusty orange, and left streets and sidewalks covered with a greenish film.

—"Menace in the Skies," *Time* (January 27, 1967), p. 49.

Cleopatra's Needle, the Egyptian obelisk brought to New York City in 1881, has been vastly more worn and scarred by its last 90 years of existence [and exposure to chemical pollutants in New York's air] than by its first 3,000.

—"The Ravaged Environment," *Newsweek* (January 26, 1970), p. 31.

Smog, a wit once remarked, is the Air Apparent. And the waste in U.S. air cripples cattle in Florida, discolors the paint on houses and automobiles in Lincoln, Maine, kills pine trees 60 miles away from Los Angeles, and ruins orchids in Texas and Illinois as well as spinach in southern California. . . .

. . . Arizona's copper industries spew tons of sulphur dioxide on Phoenix and Tucson, where it combines with automobile exhausts. In Florida, not far from Tampa and St. Petersburg, fluorides emitted from phosphate plants are absorbed by cattle; the chemicals affect the bone structure of the animals so severely that they cannot bear to stand and, instead, sink to their knees.

—"The Ravaged Environment," *Newsweek* (January 26, 1970), pp. 37F, 38.

Dirty air is shortening our lives. It contributes to respiratory disease and premature death. Air pollution is a major factor in emphysema, one of today's fastest growing causes of death. In 1958, 6,707 Americans died from the disease. In 1967, emphysema claimed 20,875, an increase of more than 200 percent.

—National Tuberculosis Association, Statistics Department.

[Dr. Bertram W. Carnow, head of a task force on the environment in Illinois:] The death rate from emphysema has doubled every five years for the last two decades. It is now the second highest cause of disability in people below the age of 65 years who apply for Social Security benefits at an annual cost in excess of $100 million.

—"The Role of Air Pollution in Chronic Obsessive Pulmonary Disease," *JAMA* (November 2, 1970), p. 895.

19

Each month 1,000 more workers are forced prematurely to retire onto Social Security rolls because of emphysema.

> —*The Effects of Air Pollution,* U.S. Public Health Service, U. S. Department of Health, Education, and Welfare (Washington, D.C., 1968).

Air pollution is a chief cause of chronic bronchitis. The number of deaths from chronic bronchitis in 1967 was more than double the number 10 years before.

> —National Tuberculosis Association, Statistics Department.

A full 90% of U.S. air pollution consists of largely invisible but potentially deadly gases. More than half of the contamination in the air over the U.S., for example, consists of colorless, odorless, carbon monoxide, most of it issuing from the exhaust pipes of automobiles, trucks and buses. . . .

Though air conditioners can effectively filter pollutant particles out of the air, the troublesome gaseous contaminants pass through unhindered. Thus city dwellers who feel that they have found sanctuary from the smog in sealed and air conditioned offices and apartments are actually in an atmosphere that may be little better than the foul air of the streets.

> —"Menace in the Skies," *Time* (January 27, 1967), pp. 49, 50.

Generally, you are as unaware of being poisoned by contaminated air as you are of breathing. Nonetheless, chemical bodies in the air can make you sick. Indeed, they can kill you.

> —Lewis, *With Every Breath You Take,* p. xv.

Many studies have linked air pollution to morbidity and mortality from pulmonary disease. Patients with severe chronic obstructive lung disease are the most susceptible to the harmful effects of air pollutants. In treating patients with these diseases, physicians should consider air pollution as a factor in illness and should treat their patients prophylactically whenever pollution levels become elevated.

> —"The Role of Air Pollution in Chronic Obstructive Pulmonary Disease," *JAMA* (November 2, 1970), p. 899.

20

. . . [Studies] indicate that: if air pollution were reduced 50 percent in our major cities, a newborn baby would have an additional three to five years life expectancy; that the same reduction in air pollution would cut death from lung disease by 25 percent and death and disease from heart and circulatory disorders by 10 to 15 percent, and that all death and diseases would be reduced annually by about 4.5 percent with a saving to the nation of at least $2 billion a year.

—Glenn Seaborg, "Do We Need Nuclear Power?," *The New York Times* (December 28, 1970), p. 31.

[Dr. Bertram W. Carnow:] The acute air pollution episodes that took place in Donora, Pa., in the Meuse valley in Belgium, and that in London in 1952 in which over 4,000 people died, suggested that certain individuals tended to be more susceptible than others to air pollutants. In particular, older people, especially with heart and lung disease, individuals with asthma, and the very young appeared to be the most affected and were the ones that became acutely ill and died.

—"The Role of Air Pollution in Chronic Obstructive Pulmonary Disease," *JAMA* (November 2, 1970), p. 895.

Though researchers have not been able to prove a direct cause-and-effect relationship between air pollution and disease, they have found that the incidence of chronic bronchitis among British mailmen who deliver mail in areas with heavy air pollution is three times as high as among mailmen who work in cleaner regions. Researchers also know that there are more deaths from chronic pulmonary disease in high-pollution areas of Buffalo than in other neighborhoods. Boston policemen working around high concentrations of carbon monoxide seem more susceptible to the common cold.

—"Menace in the Skies," *Time* (January 27, 1967), pp. 50–51.

Lung cancer is found twice as often in air polluted cities as in rural areas.

—*Needed: Clean Air*, p. 9.

[Dr. Bertram W. Carnow:] There is . . . evidence to suggest a direct relationship between the size of the city, its level of [air] pollution, and the incidence of lung cancer.

—"The Role of Air Pollution in Chronic Obstructive Pulmonary Disease," *JAMA* (November 2, 1970), p. 895.

Four independent studies have shown that longtime residence in *countries* with different degrees of air pollution was associated with different incidences of lung cancer.

—*The Effects of Air Pollution*, p. 6.

Norway, with low air pollution, has half the lung cancer of the United States.

—*Needed: Clean Air*, p. 9.

There is good evidence that air pollution contributes not only to the incidence of pulmonary cancer but to various other cancers as well.

—*Environmental Health Problems*, p. 39.

In 1968, Dr. Samuel S. Epstein told the Muskie [Senate] Subcommittee on Air and Water Pollution that "The dramatic increase in mortality from lung cancer . . . is now approaching epidemic proportions." A class of pollutants definitely identified as containing carcinogenic (cancer-producing) agents is gaseous hydrocarbons. Hydrocarbons enter the atmosphere as a result of incomplete combustion. Although industrial processes account for a substantial portion of these gases, the automobile provides more than half of all the hydrocarbons in the air we breathe.

Benzo-a-pyrene is the hydrocarbon which has been most clearly associated with cancer. It is present in cigarette smoke, and the one-pack-a-day man inhales about 3 micrograms daily. The nonsmoker in a highly polluted area takes in more benzo-a-pyrene daily than he would from a pack of cigarettes. The concentration of the pollutant is 50 million times greater in cities like New York, Chicago, or Los Angeles than in Grand Canyon National Park.

—Esposito, *Vanishing Air*, p. 12–13.

Substances floating in our atmosphere today may cause birth defects tomorrow. Such contaminants are of two types: 1. mutagens, which damage genetic intelligence and cause mutations, and 2. teratogens, which interfere with the development of the fetus, resulting in deformed babies. . . .

The most potent mutagens in the environment are ethyleneimines. These get into the air through insecticides, solid rocket fuels, emissions from textile and printing industries, and other industrial processes. Minute amounts injected into male mice caused a large number of their offspring to be deformed. Another mutagen is benzo-a-pyrene, primarily an auto by-product. This also produces malformed babies in mice, and is extremely common in urban air.

—Esposito, *Vanishing Air,* pp. 10–11.

We estimate the total annual cost that would be saved by a 50 percent reduction in air-pollution levels in major urban areas, in terms of decreased morbidity and mortality, to be $2080 million. A more relevant indication of the cost would be the estimate that 4.5 percent of all economic costs associated with morbidity and mortality would be saved [by such a reduction]. . . .

—Lester B. Lave and Eugene P. Seskin, "Air Pollution and Human Health," *Science,* Vol. 169, No. 3947 (August 21, 1970), p. 730–31.

Scientists have . . . calculated that a child born in New York City after World War II has now inhaled the pollution equivalent of smoking nine cigarettes per day every day of his life. Like those in cigarettes, some of the hydrocarbons identified in automobile exhausts have produced cancer in laboratory animals.

—"Menace in the Skies," *Time* (January 27, 1967), p. 50.

Though an hour's exposure to 1,500 parts of carbon monoxide per million parts of air can endanger a man's life, only 120 parts per million for an hour can affect his driving enough to cause an accident. And concentrations of about 100 parts per million have been found in tunnels and garages and on the streets of Chicago, Detroit, New York and London.

Assistant Surgeon General Prindle points out that a heavy cigarette smoker carries a 3% to 4% concentration of carbon monoxide in his bloodstream. Thus it is not surprising, he says, that habitual smokers are the first to turn up at hospitals during periods of extreme air pollution; carbon monoxide concentrations in their bloodstreams reach a toxic 25%–30% level before those of nonsmokers.

—"Menace in the Skies," *Time* (January 27, 1967), p. 50.

Next to autos, the worst air polluters in the nation are the power companies. . . . Despite the massive propaganda campaign waged by many utilities to prove how advanced and forward-looking they are, the industry in general is one of the most backward in the nation. Utilities are still generating power by the same general method that Thomas Alva Edison first used 86 years ago. Even nuclear power doesn't represent much of a change—only a different fuel source to produce the steam that drives the turbines—and causes quite serious polluting side effects in the process.

The utilities are the pampered darlings of our economic system. As franchised monopolies, they are protected from competition and guaranteed a comfortable profit no matter how badly they conduct their affairs. While other companies have to invest between five and 13 per cent of their net income in research and development to improve their products, the utility industry in general invests considerably less than one per cent. The lack of innovative development is the result, and the product, as far as we are concerned, is pollution.

—Ottinger, *What Every Woman Should Know*, pp. 25–26.

. . . If we were to calculate the health hazards from fossil fuel plants we should note that they are responsible for about 12 per cent by tonnage of all air pollution and that pollution contributes to about 100,000 deaths yearly (25,000 cancer of the respiratory tract, 60,000 emphysema, 3,000 bronchial asthma and an indeterminate number of cardiovascular accidents) or about 12,000 deaths annually.

It should be noted that this toll is about one third of what can happen with atomic power plants and is easily corrected if adequate pollution control devices are installed using existing technology. . . .

—David Gitlin, M.D. (letter), *The New York Times* (November 15, 1970), The Week in Review, p. 10.

Dr. Robert Karsh, Associate Attending Physician, Jewish Hospital of St. Louis, Assistant Professor of Clinical Medicine, Washington University School of Medicine . . . . : . . . Fifty-five percent of all the sulfur dioxide in our local [St. Louis] atmosphere, and throughout the United States wherever there are steam electric-power plants, comes from those installations. The control of sulfur dioxide means a fundamental change in our way of life. However, a switch to nuclear power plants merely means trading sulfur dioxide pollution for thermal water pollution and possibly for radiation pollution. So there are no easy solutions.

—"The Role of Air Pollution in Chronic Obstructive Pulmonary Disease," *JAMA* (November 2, 1970), pp. 897–98.

. . . [The] difference between 96 per cent control of soot from a large coal-burning power plant and 98 per cent control, which sounds like a trivial amount, is the difference between the surrounding residents' being exposed to one ton of soot per hour or only half a ton.

—Gladwin Hill, "Statistics Can Becloud the Pollution Picture," *The New York Times* (December 28, 1970), p. 26.

In 1969, power generation in New York City unleashed 108,300 tons of nitrogen oxides into the atmosphere. The Astoria plant alone . . . was responsible for 20,480 tons. . . . The enlargement of the Astoria plant [a plan then being considered] could conceivably double this quantity. . . .

On October 23, 1968, [Charles F.] Luce [chairman of Consolidated Edison], for the first—and . . . [possibly] only—time, acknowledged publicly the need for more research in this area [of pollution control and research]. . . . In the last five years, Con Edison has spent exactly 143,000 dollars on *all* forms of pollution research. . . . The research was actually just another aspect of the Company's public relations since it consisted of meterorological studies designed to prove that Con Ed's filth was not harming anyone.

According to *The New York Times*, Chairman Luce [receives a salary of] . . . about $200,000 dollars annually . . . more in one year than the piddling amount Con Ed spent on all air pollution research over the last five years.

—Esposito, *Vanishing Air*, pp. 216–19.

25

To coordinate the planning of power generation and transmission facilities to meet expected demand in the region from Colorado to the California coast, 23 utilities have cooperatively formed the Western Energy Supply and Transmission (WEST) Associates. . . . Under the WEST concept, two superpower plants are already operating, and three more are in early stages of construction; plans have been revealed now for a sixth. . . . These are all coal-fueled thermal plants. . . . They are some of the largest power plants in the world. . . .

The plants are located in sparsely-populated regions of New Mexico, Arizona, Nevada, and Utah—as distant as 500 miles from the areas of major consumption of the power. The impact of this complex of superpower plants on the environment of the largely desert region . . . is an issue of increasing concern to the entire country. . . .

The first of the WEST plants to go into operation was the Four Corners Plant at Fruitland, New Mexico. . . .

The plume of fly ash from the plant fills the previously clear desert air, showing little inclination to disperse. . . .

The combined emission of roughly 400 tons [of fly ash] per day from the five operating units of the Four Corners Plant make it possibly the worst single source of air pollution in the world; these emissions can be compared with the daily average production of particulates in the entire New York metropolitan region, estimated at 633 tons per day in 1966 [according to the National Air Pollution Control Administration]. In 1970 NBC [television] news pointed out that the only man-made feature on the surface of the earth which was distinguishable to astronauts returning from the moon was the Four Corners Power Plant and its plume of smoke. . . .

Impact of the WEST plants is most immediately felt by the Navajo Indian Tribe, on whose lands are the first operating and another of the three largest plants; both burn coal strip-mined from these lands. The economic impact upon the Navajos, the largest of the American nations, is impressive. . . . To them this new industry on the reservation is a means to economic elevation on a par with the white man. . . .

On the other hand, the new industry has divided the Navajo people. . . . Traditional Navajos are dismayed that the industry developments spell the end of the Navajo culture—and the loss of their identity. . . . Now, through the guise of partially improved economic conditions and because of the white man's insatiable demand for electric power, both the undesecrated landscape and the clean, azure skies are being obliterated. . . .

If strict emission standards are not imposed [New Mexico state standards are lax and even so are being exceeded by the WEST plants], the 300 tons per day of sulfur oxides emitted by the Four Corners Plant will grow to an estimated 1,365 tons per day as other plants join in. Nitrogen oxide emissions will increase similarly. . . .

Even if strict standards for fly ash emissions are imposed and enforced at all the WEST plants, the fact that extremely fine particles do form stable suspensions in air, taking weeks to disperse, makes a very real specter of the environmentalists' vision of air pollution obscuring the Grand Canyon and Lake Powell, being replenished by the haze from the power plants which are to be built on either side of Lake Powell and the Colorado River. This situation may not be avoidable with power plants of the current design, for not all the fly ash can be removed from the stacks. Prevention of it may depend upon abandonment of the pulverized fuel injection power system in favor, perhaps, of coal gasification and pre-burning purification of the gaseous fuel.

If operation of the WEST superpower plants is not to desecrate the region's major scenic, recreational, economic (tourism, agriculture, forestry) and residential values, WEST associates must abandon the attitude that the atmosphere is an infinite dump. Calculations of stack heights required for dispersal of pollutants . . . must be replaced by designs of retention and recovery processes and new approaches to coal utilization without pollution. Although WEST water contracts have traditionally stipulated that the "best commercially proven" pollution control equipment will be installed in these plants, actual practice has adhered to the attitude of minimum investment. There is no reason to expect the companies to abandon that attitude voluntarily.

—Roy Craig, "Cloud on the Desert," *Environment,* Vol. 13, No. 6 (July/August 1971), pp. 21–22, 24, 29, 33–35.

. . . [Legal] limitations now prevent the construction of most types of electric generating stations in southern California. Southern California therefore now looks to the coalfields great distances away. Extra high voltage transmission makes possible the movement of large quantities of power over long distances. And Californians, accordingly, began to look to the coalfields as far away as the four-corners area, where Arizona, New Mexico, Utah, and Colorado come together. Here there are big coal deposits, and here they found they could build large new thermal installations—750 megawatts and some of them will go to a million soon—and still achieve tremendous economies.

—Stewart L. Udall (then U.S. Secretary of the Interior), "Development of National Policy with Respect to Coal and Oil," *Proceedings-The Third National Conference on Air Pollution,* Office of Legislative and Public Affairs, National Center for Air Pollution Control (conference held on December 12–14, 1966), Public Health Service Publication No. 1649, pp. 129–30.

It has been demonstrated that the annual incidence of respiratory disease is directly proportional to the annual sulfur oxides level. As sulfur oxides levels go up, so does the incidence of disease.

It has also been found that deaths from respiratory causes are more frequent in populations exposed to higher levels of the sulfur oxides.

—*The Effects of Air Pollution,* pp. 9–10.

A flood of contamination may occur from only a single industrial source. A moderate-sized copper smelter alone emits 1,500 tons of sulfur dioxide a day; an oil refinery, 450 tons; a coal-fired plant, 300 tons. In addition, every city suffers from the vast quantities of contaminants resulting from the burning of combustibles. Each ton of fuel oil burned gives off 600 pounds of oxides of sulfur, 27 pounds of oxides of nitrogen, and 5 pounds of solids. Each ton of coal burned gives off 200 pounds of solids, 40 pounds of sulfur oxides and 8 pounds of nitrogen oxides. Each ton of refuse burned in usual incinerator methods gives off 25 pounds of solids, 4 pounds of nitrogen oxides and 2 to 8 pounds of sulfur oxides.

—Lewis, *With Every Breath You Take,* p. 43.

. . . no less than 48,000 tons of sulfur dioxide are produced each day over the United States merely from the burning of coal. In terms of volume, this amount of sulfur dioxide is enough to pollute—in vegetation-damaging concentrations—400 feet of air over 46,000 square miles, an area larger than the State of Pennsylvania.

—Lewis, *With Every Breath You Take*, p. 43.

Dust and soot are the most annoying forms of air pollution in many cities. The sources of the particulate emissions in New York City . . . [include] space heating, municipal incineration, apartment house incineration, and power generation [, which] account for about 80 percent of the 69,100 tons . . . emitted per year to the atmosphere as of November 1969.

—Merril Eisenbud, "Environmental Protection in the City of New York," *Science*, Vol. 170, No. 3959 (November 13, 1970), pp. 706–707.

With every breath, you inhale 40,000 to 70,000 dust particles. For city dwellers, that means inhaling about 1 pound 7 ounces per year. . . .

If dust were only a mess and a bother, it would be bad enough. The fact is that dust is destructive and dangerous. Dust . . . mars paint on buildings and cars . . . scratches and pits glass, . . . [reduces] visibility [,] . . . closes in airports [,] . . . [and] penetrates engines and machinery, acting like an abrasive. . . .

Worse yet, dust penetrates the human mechanism, impairing health. The hair and mucus barriers in the nasal passages are not suited to screening out particles smaller than 1/5,000th of an inch. A particle more minute than that is likely to enter the passages of the lungs. A particle 1/50,000th of an inch or smaller may enter the alveoli, the tiny sacs in the lungs where the exchange between air and blood takes place. If abnormal amounts of dust are in the air, even large particles will penetrate the lungs. In communities with dusty industries, the inhalation of dust is so great that the lungs of local residents become loaded with fairly large particles. These dust deposits make breathing more difficult. Often they lead to an enlargement of the heart, which is . . . a frequent cause of cardiac failure. . . .

Dust clogging the lungs also aggravates such respiratory infections as pneumonia and bronchitis. . . .

Allergies are induced by dust, causing severe skin eruptions, emotional disturbances, and inflammation of the eyes, nose, and throat.

29

Asthma is one of the commonest, as well as one of the most serious, of the allergic conditions provoked by dust.

—Lewis, *With Every Breath You Take*, pp. 55, 63–64.

. . . [It] must be obvious even to a nontechnical person that the coal analysis itself does no harm or damage to anyone, nor does the effluent, whatever its characteristics, at the outlet of the stack, particularly if the stack be of a height from 600 to 1200 feet.

—Philip Sporn (President, retired, American Electric Power Company, New York City). "Discussion of Preceding Three Papers," *Proceedings*, p. 146.

The fact of the matter is, of course, that stacks possess no magic power to eliminate a pollutant. They do not reduce by one gram the total amount of pollutant released to the atmosphere. They distribute it in a different way than would be true of a low-level source, but a receptor at a great distance will receive substantially the same concentrations no matter what the source height. . . . This failure to effect a widespread reduction is the essential reason for continued emphasis on restricting the total amount of emissions by those concerned with large-scale pollution problems.

—Maynard E. Smith (Leader, Meteorology Group, Brookhaven National Laboratory), "Reduction of Ambient Air Concentrations of Pollutants by Dispersion from High Stacks," *Proceedings*, pp. 154–55.

The costs to clean up the air are very low on a per citizen basis. Dust control for electric power generating plants, for example, would add only about 1 cent per month to a family's electric bill.

— *The Sources of Air Pollution and Their Control*, U.S. Public Health Service, U.S. Department of Health, Education, and Welfare (Washington, D.C., 1966), Publication No. 1548, p. 15.

A recent study [cited in *Proceedings of the New York-New Jersey Air Pollution Abatement Conference*, National Air Pollution Control Administration, Cincinnati, Ohio] indicates that dust control to a specific set of air standards in the New York [City] area would save the average citizen $50 per year in cleaning costs.

—Ralph I. Larsen, "Relating Air Pollution Effects to Concentration and Control," *Journal of the Air Pollution Control Association*, Vol. 20, No. 4 (April 1970), p. 222.

Silica and asbestos particles are dusts that have a reactive effect on the lungs. But even inert dusts, having no direct effect on lung tissue, can play a part in the development of lung cancer. . . . Chicago Medical School [investigators] demonstrated conclusively that, by carrying cancer-producing agents into the lungs, dust can be an essential factor in causing the disease. . . .

. . . [Some] cancer investigators [have theorized that] . . . dust particles encounter molecules of a carcinogenic pollutant. This meeting occurs either in the air or during the combustion process in which the carcinogen is formed. The dust adsorbs the carcinogen. More encounters, more adsorption—with a resulting high concentration of carcinogen. Someone inhales this and other dust particles. . . . The carcinogen, which has been riding on the surface of the particle, is now discharged into the lung tissue. Then, concentrated and in conjunction with other dust-carried carcinogenic substances, it may well cause a lung cancer.

—Lewis, *With Every Breath You Take*, pp. 65, 67.

Some talcum powders contain asbestos, a material that has been shown to contribute to such diseases as lung cancer. . . . [Talc] mineral beds may contain several forms of asbestos. Suspecting that this natural contamination may be carried through to the final product—talcum powder—New York's [City] Department of Air Resources sent samples of two infant talcum powders to Dr. Irving Selikoff, an authority on the dangers of asbestos inhalation. Dr. Selikoff's laboratory found that the asbestos content in the talcum powder ranged from 5 to 25 percent. Inhalation of low levels of asbestos, such as would be found in the baby powders, has not been shown to cause disease, but once asbestos particles are taken into the lung they remain there, providing a lifelong potential for the development of cancer.

—"Spectrum," *Environment*, Vol. 13, No. 7 (September 1971), p. 27.

. . . [The] overall bill in the next 34 years, to reach a goal of about one-fifth of today's fly ash emission to the atmosphere, is going to be about $400 million. This . . . can hardly be considered a tremendous cost. It amounts to about 5 cents a year per capita, and under very adverse conditions, i.e., labor costs, low sulfur fuel, etc., would amount to only 10 cents per year.

—William W. Moore, "Reduction in Ambient Air Concentration of Fly Ash—Present and Future Prospects," *Proceedings*, pp. 177–78.

A Cornell University scientist, Dr. Lamont Cole, testified before our Senate Interior Committee on my bill to authorize research into ecology. . . . Dr. Cole said: "Man is burning fossil fuel at an ever-increasing rate, and it is probable that more than half of the fuel ever burned by man has been burned in this century. One result of this is to release carbon dioxide into the atmosphere more rapidly than it can be taken up by green plants or dissolved in the oceans and eventually precipitated. . . . It appears probable that the carbon dioxide content of the atmosphere has increased by at least 10 percent since the turn of the century. . . .

". . . If we reach a point at which the rate of combustion exceeds the rate of photosynthesis, the oxygen content of the atmosphere will start to decrease."

—Gaylord Nelson (U.S. Senator from Wisconsin), "A Congressional View of the Problem," *Proceedings*, pp. 451–52.

Legal maneuvers to control smoke go back to the Britain of 1273, when Edward I issued a decree against the use of smoky Newcastle sea coal. This pointed but unsuccessful effort foreshadowed the smoke-abatement ordinances existing today in many American communities. However, even as in Edward's day, enforcement of current antismoke ordinances is spotty. Thus, while smoke and sootfall have been alleviated in some locales, they are still a major form of air pollution.

—Lewis, *With Every Breath You Take*, p. 68.

[Dr. Bertram W. Carnow:] In 14th century London, . . . it was unlawful to use soft coal because of contamination of the air.

—"The Role of Air Pollution in Chronic Obstructive Pulmonary Disease," *JAMA* (November 2, 1970), p. 894.

. . . [Fog] occurs from two to five times as often in the city as in the surroundings. Fortunately, this seems to be a reversible process. Recent clean-up campaigns have shown that, through the use of smokeless fuels, considerable lessening of the concentration of particulates, and hence of fog and the attenuation of light, can be achieved. In London, for example, with the change in heating practices, winter sunshine has increased by 70 percent in the last decade, and the winter visibilities have improved by a factor of 3 since the improvements were introduced. . . .

—*Science*, December 18, 1970, p. 1272.

In New York City during the summer, the present level of smog reduces the sunlight that reaches the ground by one-third.

—Ottinger, p. 21.

WASHINGTON, Jan. 20—. . . [According to] Senator Edmund S. Muskie of Maine, chairman of the Senate Subcommittee on Air and Water Pollution, . . . in New York [City], "planes dump one and one-half tons of pollutants per day"; . . . Los Angeles "gets almost one ton per day"; and . . . Washington [D.C.] gets 1,200 pounds. Nationally, he said 78 million pounds a year are emitted from jet engines.

—E.W. Kenworthy, "The Airlines Accept Pollution Deadline," *The New York Times* (January 21, 1970), p. 26.

In Rumford, Maine; Lewiston, Idaho; and scores of small towns like them, the [pulp and paper] mill maintains a virtual monopoly on employment. The monopoly is perpetuated by the stink. Businessmen in search of a rural setting for a new electronics or assembly plant look elsewhere. . . .

. . . The constant stench, the nausea, vomiting, insomnia, headaches, increased irritability, mental stress, respiratory ailments, allergies, the chipping and blackening of paint, and the disastrous decline in property values become more difficult to shrug off. Some people are even beginning to wonder about the long-term effects of kraft mill odor on mental health, learning capacity, and productivity. Hydrogen sulfide, the nerve-paralyzing gas, responsible for most of the odor, is being sniffed with increasing alarm. A report [*Air Pollution Aspects of*

33

Hydrogen Sulfide] prepared for NAPCA by Litton Industries notes, "Hydrogen sulfide is highly toxic to humans, and at [high] concentrations . . . quickly causes death by paralysis of the respiratory system. At lower concentrations, hydrogen sulfide may cause conjunctivitis with reddening and lachrymal secretion, respiratory tract irritation, psychic changes, pulmonary edema, damaged heart muscle, disturbed equilibrium, nerve paralysis, spasms, unconsciousness and circulatory collapse." The physiological effects of continuous exposure to very low levels have never been thoroughly studied.

—Esposito, *Vanishing Air,* pp. 130–31.

In amounts emitted by industrial plants in several sections of the country, fluorides cause eye irritations, nosebleeds, inflammations of the respiratory tract, and severe difficulties in breathing. To judge from sufferings of cattle that have been exposed to fluorides, the chemicals are also capable of wearing away teeth and of malforming bones and joints.

Fluorides are emitted by steel mills, aluminum plants, brick and tile works, and manufacturers of artificial fertilizer. . . .

. . . The fluorides are extremely poisonous to plants. In large areas, shrubbery has withered away. Commercial gladiolus growing has suffered extensively. Some 25,000 acres of citrus groves have been destroyed.

—Lewis, *With Every Breath You Take,* p. 110.

"It's cheaper to pay claims than it is to control fluorides." These are the words of an executive of the Reynolds Metals Company, quoted in an opinion written by a federal appeals court judge [Reynolds Metals v. Lampert, 324 F. 2d 465, 466 (9th cir. 1963)].

—Esposito, *Vanishing Air,* p. 69.

In semi-rural Florida, east of Tampa, large amounts of fluorides emitted from phosphate plants have rained down on nearby citrus groves, ranches and gladiolus farms. Orange and lemon trees that absorbed the fluorides produced smaller yields, and gladioli turned brown and died. A national air-pollution symposium reported that cattle grazing on

34

grass that was contaminated with fluorides developed uneven teeth that hindered chewing and joints so swollen that many of the animals could not stand. Fluorides have also etched windowpanes, giving them the frosted appearance of a light bulb.

—"Menace in the Skies," *Time* (January 27, 1967), p. 50.

Despite the celebrated alleged clean-ups in cities like Pittsburgh and St. Louis, the air of urban America is more dangerous today than ever before. It may not be as visible, but our polluted air today is a greater hazard to health and a greater destroyer of property.

—William F. Ryan (then U. S. Representative 20th District, New York), "A Congressional View of the Problem," *Proceedings*, p. 343.

Air pollution has caused great damage and destruction to vegetation, and now places very real restrictions on the types of vegetation that may be raised in many areas of the country. For example:

—Smog in California has made it impossible to raise orchids, and the growers have had to relocate.

—In New Jersey—the Garden State—pollution injury to vegetation has been observed in every single county, and damage has been reported to at least 36 commercial crops (spinach, endive, etc.).

—Orange trees in Florida have been severely damaged, causing growers to relocate.

—*The Effects of Air Pollution*, p. 14.

Virtually every urban area in the nation now experiences damage to vegetation from air pollution, and many rural areas that once were thought to be safely removed from pollution sources are now experiencing crop injury.

—*The Effects of Air Pollution*, p. 14–15.

Scientists are certain that the ozone and PAN [peroxyacyl nitrate] in Los Angeles smogs have caused the serious decline in the citrus and salad crops in the area.

—"Menace in the Skies," *Time* (January 27, 1967), p. 50.

Each year the U.S. alone paves over 1,000,000 acres of oxygen-producing trees.

—"Fighting to Save the Earth from Man," *Time* (February 2, 1970), pp. 62.

Almost every state now turns in reports of plant damage from air pollution. One national estimate of injury to all types of vegetation is as high as half a billion dollars annually.

A survey made in New York last fall of woody plant damage caused by air pollution showed that many familiar trees and shrubs were showing signs of injury. Lilacs, beeches, lindens, dogwood, ginko and white pine foliage had flecking, scorch patterns and browning on the underside of the leaves. The survey was conducted in Central and Prospect Parks and in the Brooklyn Botanic Garden.

—Joan Lee Faust "... But Air Pollution Threatens," *The New York Times* (October 25, 1970), Arts and Leisure section, p. 39.

. . . Trees . . . happen to be an important part of this planet's life-support system.

Those little green bodies in the leaves, called chloroplasts, which give the foliage its green color, are vital manufacturing plants. The leaves utilize carbon dioxide combined with water to manufacture the trees' food supply which is stored in a form of starch. The "exhaust" from this vital photosynthesis process is oxygen and the energy from the sun makes the whole system work.

When air pollutants contaminate this process, many trees are in trouble. A leaf's air intake is through tiny pores called stomates, most of which are located on the surface. When polluted air enters leaves of susceptible trees, the plant chlorophyl is often destroyed, the photosynthesis process is disrupted and the plant is either stunted, chlorotic (yellowed) or in severe cases of long exposure . . . dead.

—Joan Lee Faust, "...But Air Pollution Threatens," *The New York Times* (October 25, 1970), p. 39.

The cost to the United States of dirty air is more than $12 billion a year.

—annual crop damage alone is estimated at $500 million.

—incomplete combustion in factories and power plants wastes $300 million worth of sulfur.

—it is estimated that air pollution in some cities—such as Chicago—reduces sunlight by 40 percent, causing higher lighting bills.

—*Needed: Clean Air,* pp. 6–7.

. . . in terms of property destruction alone, air pollution inflicts more damage on New York City in any given year than all the fires and all the crimes combined. It probably kills more people too.

—Esposito, *Vanishing Air,* p. 210.

The World Health Organization's expert committee to set up the air-quality criteria . . . worked out a set of general guides for air pollution assessment. . . . In all categories of pollutants, standards have been set to determine the tolerable level of admixtures in the air.

Further studies are being continued to determine the relation between the concentration of pollutants, the duration of exposure, and the effect upon man's health. So far, six countries have adopted criteria for air acceptibility; these are the US, the USSR, Romania, Poland, Czechoslovakia, and the Federal Republic of Germany. WHO urges other countries to adopt air pollution criteria and to institute measures for cleaning up the air and the whole environment.

—"What Standards for Air Quality," JAMA, Vol. 214, No. 9 (November 30, 1970), p. 1717.

Despite the hazards that air pollution holds, contaminating the atmosphere is a routine part of everyday life. In few other ways do men so heedlessly and systematically add to their own injury. And yet, since air pollution is as ordinary as are the human activities that produce it, it is easy to lose sight of air pollution's magnitude by dint of its familiarity.

—Lewis, *With Every Breath You Take,* p. 37.

Atmospheric surveillance is necessary in order to identify airborne pollutants, to establish ambient concentrations of these pollutants, and to record their trends and patterns. . . .

States have the primary responsibility for atmospheric surveillance. Surveillance systems are usually established on a city or regional basis. The federal monitoring system is to provide a base of uniform data for verification of data from the various agencies and to quantify pollutants that are difficult or expensive to measure.

Presently, the operation of most of the devices and analyzers used for measuring air pollutants is based on wet chemical methods. New techniques are needed in which solid-state or advanced sensing techniques that are based on the physical or physiochemical properties of pollutants are used. A number of new instruments are presently being developed by NAPCA [National Air Pollution Control Administration]. In addition, NAPCA has automated and computer-interfaced some of its more sophisticated laboratory and field instrumentation.

—Morgan, Ozolins, and Tabor, "Air Pollution Surveillance Systems," *Science* (October 16, 1970), pp. 295–96.

. . . The unwholesome mess that U.S. citizens and corporations spew into that great sewer in the sky costs them dearly—$11 billion a year in property damage alone, according to the department of Health, Education and Welfare. Air pollutants abrade, corrode, tarnish, soil, erode, crack, weaken and discolor materials of all varieties. Steel corrodes from two to four times as fast in urban and industrial regions as in rural areas, where much less sulphur-bearing coal and oil are burned. The erosion of some stone statuary and buildings is also greatly speeded by high concentrations of sulphur oxides.

Heavy fallout of pollution particles in metropolitan areas deposits layers of grime on automobiles, clothing, buildings, and windows; it adds about $600 per year in washing, cleaning, repairing and repainting bills to the budget of a family with two or three children in New York City, according to a study made by Irving Michelson, a consultant in environmental health and safety.

—"Menace in the Skies," *Time* (January 27, 1967), p. 50.

The economic loss in large urban areas [due to air pollution] is thought to average $65 per person per year, but there have been no studies as to how these costs can be apportioned among the various sources of air pollution.

—Eisenbud, "Environmental Protection in the City of New York," *Science* (November 13, 1970), p. 708.

Pittsburgh, Pennsylvania, once known as the Smoky City, has reduced its smoke by an amazing 84 per cent since World War II. The success came through cooperative community action. Householders, industry, railroads and shipping lines, and coal mines, all voluntarily changed their habits in order to reduce smoke-production. The total investment in fuel change-over, installation of cleaning devices and process changes to clean the air since World War II has amounted to over $380,000,000, 25 percent of which was paid by home-owners and the rest by industry.

The annual estimated personal savings in laundry bills (not to mention health), amounted to $41 million. A smoke-control ordinance was passed in 1941 and put into effect after the War. Another was passed in 1949. By 1955 there was a reduction of 96.6 per cent in heavy smoke and of 88.8 per cent in total smoke since 1946. Visibility, which used to be barely across the street, had been extended to 10 miles on most days by 1970. Their battle against air pollution is not over: attention is now turning to the invisible pollutants, such as carbon monoxide and sulphur dioxide.

 —*UNESCO Courier.*

Simon Mencher, until recently Deputy Commissioner of the [New York City] Department of Air Resources, . . . [said,] ". . . we get 32,000 complaints each year. We get to about 15 per cent of them. If we tried to answer them all, we wouldn't be able to do anything else. . . ."

 —Esposito, *Vanishing Air,* pp. 209–10.

New York [City] has only about seventy-five regular air pollution inspectors as compared with 200 sanitation inspectors and 1,000 building inspectors.

 —"Earth Watch," *Saturday Review* (November 7, 1970), p. 70.

The measures that must be adopted in New York City to implement the present provisions of the air pollution control law will cost about $500 million by about 1972. If the economic losses due to air pollution are as high as has been estimated, this is obviously a good investment, since the city's 8 million residents would receive a return on their investment of more than 100 percent per year, assuming the estimated economic loss to be $65 per capita [per year].

—Eisenbud, "Environmental Protection in the City of New York," *Science* (November 13, 1970), p. 708.

Sulphur dioxide [in the air] . . . has been reduced markedly here [New York City] by restricting the sulphur content of fuel that may be used for heating and power generation. . . .

The Mayor announced that, as of Aug. 18, there already had been 24 "good" days [in 1971], according to the city's daily air pollution control index, while in all of 1969 and 1970 there had been no "good" days at all.

The city's air pollution index—which runs on a scale from "good" to "acceptable" and "unsatisfactory" to "unhealthy,"—depends heavily on the concentration of sulphur dioxide in the air.

—David Bird, "Rise in Dirt Particles Found in City's Air," *The New York Times* (September 20, 1971), p. 51.

Despite strict new controls on air pollution, more particles of dirt are in New York City's air than last year, the latest statistics indicate. . . . In July [1971] . . . 76 per cent of the citywide samples exceeded . . . [the new Federal standards that, as of 1975, will allow no more than 75 micrograms of particulates per cubic meter of air]. In the preceding 12 months, 73 per cent of the samples were above that mark.

Manhattan had the dirtiest air, with 92 per cent of the samples above the Federal mean in July. Again the figure was lower—86 per cent—over the previous 12 months.

The peak 24-hour readings around the city also are higher. As of the end of July, the highest reading, which was taken in Manhattan, was 581 micrograms per cubic meter. A year ago that peak was only 407. . . .

Particles of dirt in the city's air come from every conceivable source—bits of rubber tires and asbestos brake lining from automobiles, cement and plaster dust from construction and demolition sites, soot from chimneys that may vent anything from simple furnaces or plants making complex plastic compounds.

It is because the particles come in such variety here ... [according to a Federal official], "that the solution is not as clear-cut as, say, reducing sulphur in oil and coal to cut down on sulphur dioxide."

—Bird, "Rise in Dirt Particles Found in City's Air, *The New York Times* (September 20, 1971), p. 51.

3

Automobile Pollution

✳

. . . Today, there is no part of the environment that that infernal vehicle, the automobile, does not despoil. Its internal combustion engine pollutes the air. Wrecked, abandoned, or simply replaced by a newer model, its hulks litter country fields, rust along stream and lake banks, clutter city alleys. . . .

The automobile must bear a good share of the blame for many present troubles. It has contributed greatly to urban sprawl, inner-city decay, air and water pollution, contamination of soil and plant life, noise, unsightliness . . .[and] "near-toxic levels" of lead in American air, soil, and water. . . .

. . . [were] it not for the automobile, the petroleum industry would not be polluting the nation's rivers and air, and, through tanker spills, the world's oceans. . . . Nor would the steel mills have so darkened the skies over many towns and cities. Nor would the noise level from city traffic have risen to decibels almost unbearable to the human ear and nervous system.

—William E. Small, *Third Pollution:The National Problem of Solid Waste Disposal* (Praeger, 1971), pp. 76–79.

Today, the automobile and its internal combustion engine are responsible for about 60 per cent of the poisonous filth in our air. In some metropolitan areas the auto is the source of as much as 80 per cent of the pollution.

—Ottinger, *What Every Woman Should Know*, p. 21.

By the year 2000 the number of cars can be expected to have quadrupled—and will burn 160 billion gallons of gasoline each year.

—*Environmental Health Problems*, p. 8.

45

The number of motor vehicles in this country increases *twice as fast* as the number of people.

—*Needed: Clean Air*, p. 11.

Some 90 million motor vehicles currently being driven in the United States are responsible, in large part, for polluting our air. Of these, 99 percent burn gasoline—some 40 billion gallons a year—with pollution from exhaust pipe, crank case, carburetor, and gas tank.

The emissions break down as follows:
—carbon monoxide: 66 million tons
—sulfur and nitrogen gases: 7 million tons
—hydrocarbons: 12 million tons
—particulates: 1 million tons

TOTAL: 86 million tons of automobile wastes polluted our air in 1969.

—*Needed: Clean Air*, p. 10.

Most physicians understand that the internal combustion engine gives off carbon monoxide, hydrocarbons, and other gases, but very few realize that *the automobile is the most important single source of air pollution in the United States today!* And it should be emphasized that this is not just a matter of dirty, smelly sun-hiding air, but is a serious health hazard.

—"The Price of Automobiles," *JAMA*, Vol. 214, No. 9 (August 31, 1970), p. 1419.

. . . [At] least 250,000 tons of carbon monoxide are discharged from motor vehicles each day in the United States. This daily output of a poison gas is enough to pollute, at a body-damaging level, 400 feet of air over a 20,000-square-mile area. Covering the combined areas of Massachusetts, Connecticut, and New Jersey, that concentration of carbon monoxide would alter every person's bodily functions enough to cause chronic disease.

—Lewis, *With Every Breath You Take*, pp. 43–44.

Carbon monoxide is one of the most common pollutants in urban air. When this poisonous gas enters the bloodstream, it replaces the oxygen needed to carry on the body's metabolism.

At high concentrations it kills quickly.

—*The Effects of Air Pollution*, p. 8.

At approximately 100 parts of carbon monoxide for every million parts of air most people experience dizziness, headache, lassitude, and other symptons of poisoning.

Concentrations higher than this occur in tunnels, in garages, or behind automobiles, i.e. in traffic.

—*The Effects of Air Pollution*, p. 8.

Driving a typical American car in city traffic for an hour pours a pound or more of carbon monoxide into the air—and there are enough cars, trucks, and buses driven in New York City *every workday* to make 8 million pounds of it.

—*Can Man Survive*, Official Publication of the Centennial 1869–1969, The American Museum of Natural History (New York, 1969), p. 4.

A recent study of parking garages in Rochester, New York revealed CO [carbon monoxide] concentrations of 300 parts per million (ppm); parking attendants were found to have concentrations of up to 20 per cent CO in their blood after only two hours of work. The effects of CO are well-documented. Concentrations of 30 per cent cause serious toxic effects; concentrations of 70 per cent in hemoglobin are invariably fatal. New York State has pegged the maximum acceptable CO concentration in the air at 30 ppm. By Navy standards, that is three times too high. Garages aren't the only danger areas. In open-air toll plazas in New York City, CO levels reach 132 ppm; in tunnels, which have extensive ventilating systems, the levels reach 118 ppm.

—Ottinger, *What Every Woman Should Know*, p. 21.

During peak weekday traffic periods, CO [carbon dioxide] levels at 45th Street and Lexington Avenue . . . often reach 25 ppm [parts per million] or two and one-half times the recommended federal standard. These

47

measurements do not reflect the concentrations on the *inside* of automobiles. "I wouldn't be surprised," [said] . . . Dr. Edward F. Ferrand, Director of Technical Services for the [New York City] Department of Air Resources, "if the average taxi driver in rush hour traffic was breathing a hundred, two hundred, maybe two hundred-fifty parts per million of CO."

—Esposito, *Vanishing Air,* p. 220.

"It appears that our city is conducting a large-scale uncontrolled experiment to determine whether low levels of all these chemicals given simultaneously are harmful to the tunnel workers. An experiment of this kind would be considered unethical in the laboratory, and is unnecessary in our society." So wrote [in 1966] the New York Scientists' Committee for Public Information, a private nonprofit group of scientists and doctors, after studying working conditions at the Queens-Midtown and Brooklyn-Battery Tunnels. The tunnel workers, they found, were being exposed to dangerous levels of such automotive-produced pollution as carbon monoxide, lead, suspended particulates, benzo-a-pyrene, asbestos, and oxides of nitrogen. In almost every instance, the levels of contamination in the toll booths and in the tunnels far exceeded established health threshold levels. For example, the federal government recommends that concentrations of particulate matter should not exceed 80 micrograms per cubic meter. . . . The reported average concentration at the Brooklyn-Battery Tunnel is 904 . . . [micrograms per cubic meter]. A recent study by the prestigious National Academy of Sciences and the National Academy of Engineering indicates that the risk of increased deaths among persons with cardiovascular diseases increases significantly when ambient carbon monoxide levels reach 10 parts per million. By that standard, the situation in New York's tunnels and bridges comes close to catastrophic. During a sampling period, [it was] . . . found that maximum hourly averages for CO reached the following levels:

Verrazano Bridge, Lane No. 11	86 ppm
Triborough Bridge, Lane No. 9	128 ppm
Queens-Midtown Tunnel, Lane No. 7	132 ppm
Brooklyn-Battery Tunnel, Lane No. 7	64 ppm

Twenty-four hour averages at all these locations generally exceeded 20 ppm and sometimes 30 ppm.

—Esposito, *Vanishing Air*, pp. 219–20.

. . . [A] popular misconception is that the automobile is the main polluter because its emissions are greater in quantity than any other source of air pollution. Thus in New York City in 1967 it was estimated that automobiles discharged 1.7 million tons of CO [carbon monoxide] per year. The next largest pollutant was SO_2 [sulfur dioxide], . . . being emitted at a rate of 828,000 tons per year. However, SO_2 is far more noxious than CO, for which the tentative air quality criterion is 15 ppm [parts per million] in New York State, as compared to about 0.1 ppm for SO_2. Thus the SO_2 emissions, though only about 48 percent of the CO emissions, are far more significant because its permissible concentration is less than 1 percent of that for CO.

—Eisebud, "Environmental Protection in the City of New York," *Science* (November 13, 1970), p. 707.

A test reported by the British magazine *Which?* (the counterpart of the American *Consumer Reports*) [in November 1969] showed that exposure to automotive fumes reduced the ability to respond to vigilance tests, the ability to add numbers quickly and accurately, the ability to comprehend sentences quickly, and the ability to make coordinated muscle response movements. "The drop in performance," the magazine reported, "is about as bad as it would be with people who had lost a night's sleep."

—Esposito, *Vanishing Air*, pp. 18–19.

In Tokyo, where smog warnings were issued on 154 days last year [1966], policemen in ten heavily polluted districts return to the station house to breathe pure oxygen after each half-hour stint on traffic duty in order to counteract the effects of breathing excessive amounts of carbon dioxide.

—"Menace in the Skies," *Time* (January 27, 1967), pp. 48–49.

A traffic study made in 1907 shows that horse-drawn vehicles in New York [City] moved at an average speed of 11.5 miles per hour. Today [1970], automobiles crawl at the average daytime rate of six miles per hour.

—Martin Gellen, "The Making of a Pollution-Industrial Complex," *Ramparts* (May 1970), p. 24.

The horse-drawn brewery days that were once so much a part of the Munich, Germany scene are disappearing, reports Medical World News (April 30). The colorful sight of the horses is vanishing, not because the horses slow down motorized traffic, but because fumes from cars and trucks are making the horses sick.

—"Spectrum," *Environment*, Vol. 13, No. 6 (July/August 1971), p. 28.

The heavy automobile traffic in the area [of the Philadelphia Zoo] has taken its toll of the zoo's residents. In 1964 Senator Edmund S. Muskie's Subcommittee was told of a sixty-two year study of mammal and bird deaths at the zoo. Autopsies of thousands of animals showed that since 1902 there had been a sixfold increase in lung cancer deaths among nine families of mammals and five families of birds.

—Esposito, *Vanishing Air*, p. 13.

The streets [of Rome, Italy] are almost permanently choked with cars. . . .

. . . [The] car is so ubiquitous that pollution from exhaust fumes has corroded monuments and caused trees to shrivel and die.

—Paul Hofmann, "After a Century as Italy's Capital, the Eternal City Suffers Modern Agonies," *The New York Times* (September 21, 1970), p. 20.

More than 100,000 electrically propelled vehicles are in operation in Great Britain already.

—Small, *Third Pollution*, p. 88.

Federal controls now require the limitation of emissions on new diesel- and gasoline-powered automobiles, buses, and trucks. Motor vehicles will remain a major polluting source for years to come, however, even with present-day controls, because (1) only new vehicles are controlled; (2) only crankcase emissions are completely eliminated, even theoretically, and, of exhaust emissions, only a portion of the hydrocarbons and carbon monoxide is removed; (3) so far, the controlling devices do not seem to be meeting even the legal requirements; and (4) methods of controlling the nitrogen oxides are still being researched.

—National Tuberculosis and Respiratory Disease Association, *Air Pollution Primer* (New York: The Association, 1969), p. 25.

Admittedly, restricting the mobility of our automobile-oriented society is a strong demand, but it is typical of the kind of restrictions we are going to have to learn to live with as we place increasing strain upon the inflexible limitations of our environment.

—Louis J. Fuller, "Concluding Remarks," (County Air Pollution Control Officer, Los Angeles), *Proceedings*, p. 459.

. . . [The] results of tests on a petrol [gasoline] engine carried out at the Warren Spring Laboratory (unpublished report RR/17/59) . . . suggest that an increase in air: fuel ratio from the rich mixture that would give maximum power to the lean mixture that would give maximum economy produces a tenfold increase in the emission of oxides of nitrogen. It therefore seems probable that the more efficient use of petrol, while reducing the emission of carbon monoxide and unburnt hydrocarbons, would cause a significant increase in the amounts of a pollutant which cannot be removed by oxidation in the exhaust system.

—A. L. Harris (letter), *New Scientist*, Vol. 46, No. 700 (May 7, 1970), pp. 300–301.

Fully aware of the pressure to reform, Detroit will introduce 1971 models that exhale only 37% as much carbon monoxide as did 1960 models. To achieve this, however, requires increased engine heat, which in turn will increase the nitrogen oxide emissions. And nitrogen oxides are particularly dangerous: under sunlight, they react with waste hydrocarbons from gasoline to form PAN (peroxyacl nitrate), along with ozone, the most toxic element in smog.

—"Fighting to Save the Earth from Man," *Time* (February 2, 1970), p. 59.

Even if the [anti-pollution] devices [on cars] work perfectly, however, they cannot keep pace with the rapid growth of Los Angeles' auto population—which is expected to increase by another 2,000,000 vehicles by 1980. "Even if by then the average motor vehicle is producing only one-half the pollution of today's average car," says County Air Pollution Control Officer Louis Fuller, "motor-vehicle pollution will be greater than it is now."

—"Menace in the Skies," *Time* (January 27, 1967), p. 51.

Tetraethyl lead is put into most gas[oline] to improve performance, and as a result auto exhausts are dumping about 300,000 tons of lead into our atmosphere each year. . . . Studies conducted by Dr. Henry A. Schroeder at the Trace Element Laboratory of Dartmouth Medical School indicate how very dangerous the lead from leaded gasoline is. Test animals fed lead in amounts equal to that now taken in by humans were found to have their life spans shortened by some 20 per cent. In addition, they showed reduced fertility and increases in infant mortality and birth malformations. Other tests taken along a moderately traveled highway showed that the lead content in the grass was enough to cause abortions in grazing cattle. Not only is the lead itself poisonous, but it quickly destroys the effectiveness of the new catalytic mufflers that are used on new cars to control other of forms of pollution.

—Ottinger, *What Every Woman Needs to Know*, pp. 23–24.

There is growing evidence that lead air pollution caused by automobiles is one of the most critical problems facing the health of urban populations.

Scientists say that breathing in microscopic particles of lead puts the toxic heavy metal into the bloodstream, where it attacks the brain, nervous system and bone structure. Children are thought to be more susceptible to lead than adults.

—James M. Staples, "Lead Particles in Air Seen as Peril to Brain, Blood and Bones," *The* (Newark, N. J.) *Evening News* (April 29, 1971), p. 26.

In the U.S. in 1968 alone, more than five hundred million pounds of lead were used as antiknock additives during this single year. About ten percent of this amount, i.e., fifty million pounds of lead, were emitted into the ambient atmosphere within the state of California; and the majority of these lead pollutants were discharged in densely populated Southern California. About half the lead in gasoline is introduced into the atmosphere as long-lived finely divided aerosols. Since the advent of leaded gasoline, a cumulative amount of more than seven billion pounds of lead have been marketed and consumed as antiknock additives in the U.S.

> —Tsaihwa J. Chow and John L. Earl, "Trend of Increasing Lead Aerosols in the Atmosphere," *Symposium on Geochemistry of Atmospheric Constituents* (annual meeting of the American Chemical Society, Houston, Texas, February 25, 1970), p. 22.

. . . [Researchers] at New York Medical College (NYMC) have discovered that a large proportion of the animals at Staten Island Zoo suffer from lead poisoning. And while some of the lead in the animals' bodies may have come from paint in their cages, the major source appears to be atmospheric contamination. . . .

Significantly, the animals kept in outdoor cages, including those in cages without paint, showed the highest levels of lead in their bodies. Even the carcasses of dead mice found inside and outside the zoo buildings were loaded with lead.

. . . The same doctors made a preliminary investigation of animals in the Bronx Zoo and turned up the same problem, although fewer animals seem to be affected.

> —Robert J. Bazell, "Lead Poisoning: Zoo Animals May Be the First Victims," *Science*, Vol. 173, No. 3992 (July 9, 1971), pp. 130–31.

In Los Angeles it is always more comfortable to ignore the [air] pollution or deny the seriousness of the threat than to face the deeper issues raised by its foul existence. Thus, a 1970 ballot proposal that would have allowed local governments to use a fixed percentage of gasoline tax revenues for research, and for a pilot study of mass transit and other alternatives to the automobile, was soundly defeated by southern California. A highly financed propaganda barrage against the plan was put on by the Southern California Auto Club in combination with oil, concrete, and highway interests.

> —Ira J. Winn, "Greetings from Los Angeles," *Natural History*, Vol. LXXX, No. 8 (October 1971), p. 16.

On an average day, the 7 million people of Los Angeles County pump about 26 million pounds of smoke and soot into the air, . . . 3.2 pounds of smog [a day] for every man, woman, and child in the area.

> —Ira J. Winn, "Greetings from Los Angeles," *Natural History* (October 1971), pp. 16, 18.

Now, as you drive along the highway in a modern American car, the engine of the car consumes well over a thousand times as much oxygen as do you. To carry off the exhaust gases, and dilute them to harmless concentrations, requires from 5 to 10 million times as much air as the driver. In other words, just one automobile, moving along a Los Angeles County Freeway, needs as much air to disperse its waste products as do all the people in the county for breathing. [According to a subsequent letter to this editor, Prof. Leighton wrote "in the nine years since the paper was written, automobile exhaust emissions have been reduced, but the methods used to reduce them have caused the oxygen consumption per automobile to increase, and still further increases are in prospect."]

> —Philip A. Leighton, "Man and Air in California." Paper presented at the Statewide Conference on Man in California, 1980s, on Jan. 27, 1964.

When the first horseless carriage necessitated the removal of a single tree, the rape of the land by the automobile began, and it has proceeded at an accelerating pace since. But what's a tree? Mayor Daley of Chicago said in answer to that question when the public tried desperately to save the destruction of some trees to make room for a roadway, "You can't stop progress." And Mr. Ronald Reagan, the hero of "Death Valley Days," shortly before he was elected Governor of California, stated in connection with the drive to save the redwoods, "If you've seen one tree, you've seen them all." It was, doubtless, the kind of remark that helped to get him elected. Only God, it has been said, can make a tree. But, of course, man can make cars much faster than God is able to make trees, or so it would appear. For the trees vanish as the cars increase. In the folly that leads him to perpetrate such disasters, man fails to perceive that there is a vital connection, affecting his own welfare, between the number of trees and the number of cars. For it is mainly our leafy trees which, by photosynthesis, give us our oxygen. Hence, when we kill trees, we reduce our sources of oxygen supply, for with the exhausts from our cars and the pollutants we empty into the air from other sources, we are depositing in the atmosphere a layer of carbon which cuts down the necessary sunlight and which, together with the already reduced foliage available, further reduces the process of photosynthesis. Instead of cutting down trees, we should be planting them. For every automobile put on the road there should be 10 trees planted; for every truck, 100 trees planted; and for every jet, 1,000 trees planted. . . .

As a consequence of the pollutants we put into the air in these ways plants wilt, their lower or under surfaces coated and glazed with a silvery sheen . . .; livestock sickens, and meat and dairy products are affected; stone, paint, and mortar are eaten away from our buildings, monuments, and bridges; and metal is corroded. And as for ourselves, well, there are so many of us that we behave as if *we* . . . were expendable. What these poisons in the air do to our eyes, mucous membranes, throats, and lungs, not to mention other organs, is damaging enough . . . to constitute a serious threat to the continuing health of the nation.

—Adapted by Ashley Montagu from his book *The American Way of Life* (New York: Putnam's, 1967), pp. 320–21.

There are some 6,000 communities in the United States which are seriously affected by atmospheric pollution. The U. S. Public Health Service has estimated that in various ways this pollution costs the American people the staggering sum of 11,000,000,000 dollars a year. And most of this pollution has its source in automobiles. It has been estimated that every 1,000 automobiles operating in an urban community discharge daily into the atmosphere 3.2 tons of carbon monoxide, 400 to 800 pounds of hydrocarbon gases, 100 to 300 pounds of nitrous oxides, and smaller amounts of sulfur and other irritants. Additional damaging products of the disastrous automobile, scarcely ever mentioned, are the solid particles, some so small they cannot be seen by the naked eye, such as bits of pulverized rock, ground metal filings, particles of rubber, residues of carbon, ash, lead, and carbohydrates. Then there are the droplets of oil, grease, and tar that drift suspended in air currents. . . .

—Montagu, *The American Way of Life*, pp. 321–22.

LA JOLLA, Calif., Dec. 26—Some of the lead pollutant from automobile exhausts may be finding its way into man's body by way of the fish he eats, according to a study underway here at the Scripps Institution of Oceanography.

Dr. T. J. Chow, marine chemist said that . . . sea bass caught off the southern California coast near smog-plagued Los Angeles showed an average content of 22 parts of lead for each million parts of liver tissue — two to three times the normal amount. . . .

Dr. Chow's certainty that the incidence of lead in the livers of fish would be traced principally to automobile emissions rests largely on isotopic examinations of the lead and on his findings that airborne lead from such emissions appears to be polluting waters 200 miles or more offshore and to depths of 30,000 feet.

—"Lead is Studied in Coastal Fish," *The New York Times* (December 27, 1970), p. 23.

. . . [In] 1966 [according to Dr. T. J. Chow of the Scripps Institution of Oceanography], it was established that water 200 miles off the California coast contained .36 micrograms of lead for each liter, or an amount 18 times greater than in the middle of the Mediterranean and 50 times greater than in the Atlantic 15 miles upwind from Bermuda.

"Before lead was first mined around 2,500 B.C. we have reason to believe there was only about .015 micrograms of lead in a liter of ocean water," he said. "So you can see how the danger is piling up."

—"Lead is Studied in Coastal Fish," *The New York Times* (December 27, 1970), p. 23.

There is vast disagreement among experts on whether lead-free gasoline is better or worse in the long run for people around heavy traffic. One faction believes people will be better off because of less lead in the air. The other camp says lead-free gas has so many other kinds of additives that it's probably worse.

—James M. Staples, "Lead Particles in Air Seen as Peril to Brain, Blood and Bones," *The* (Newark, N. J.) *Evening News* (April 29, 1971), p. 26.

Our measurement of lead in the oldest ice layer at Camp Century [in northwestern Greenland] at 1753 A.D. corresponds to the beginning of the European Industrial Revolution (in production terms), and it can be seen that lead concentrations there at this date are already more than twenty-five times higher than natural levels. . . . Lead concentrations apparently tripled in Camp Century snows during the half-century 1753–1815. They seem to double again during the following century, 1815–1933. . . . During the next three decades, 1933–1965, lead concentrations rose abruptly by a factor of about three. Today, lead concentrations in Camp Century snows are well over five hundred times above natural levels.

> —M. Murozumi, Tsaihwa J. Chow, and C. Patterson, "Chemical Concentrations of Pollutant Lead Aerosols, Terrestrial Dusts and Sea Salts in the Greenland and Antarctic Snow Strata," *Geochimica et Cosmochimica Acta*, Vol. 33 (1969), pp. 1247–1294.

Lead isn't the only problem. A compound of nickel carbonyl that results from the burning of petroleum and diesel fuels has been shown to cause lung cancer; and current uses of these fuels are dumping an estimated $110 million of this compound into our air each year.

> —Ottinger, *What Every Woman Should Know*, p. 24.

The automobile bombards us with odors and noises. It covers our highways and countryside with oil and grease, blown-out tires and rubber scraps, burnt-out mufflers and tailpipes, plus the unsightly bottles and other trash thrown out by unthinking drivers and passengers. Finally, the automobile fills huge junk yards, or worse, remains as a deserted, decaying hulk at the side of the road. The cost of cleanup and disposal has become so great that serious proposals are being made to add at least $25 to the cost of the automobile to provide for its proper burial.

> —"The Price of Automobiles," *JAMA* (August 31, 1970), p. 1419.

No part of the nation is now without overflowing auto graveyards. By 1975, the retirement rate of cars will reach 8 million a year. By 1980, the total number of vehicles on the roads will be above 120 million.

. . . Where will all the wrecked cars go? . . .

. . . [There has been a] rapid increase of automobile graveyards, which now number about 8,000.

—Small, *Third Pollution*, p. 79.

New York City picks up about 30,000 cars abandoned on its streets each year. [There] were about 830,000 motor vehicles abandoned in the United States in 1965, on public and private property—about two a minute—or well over 10 percent of the total cars retired that year.

—Small, *Third Pollution*, p. 82.

The auto wrecking and scrap industries are multibillion-dollar enterprises in the United States. Because of new technologies and the introduction of new materials, however, the fraction of salvageable waste materials and the demand for scrap are diminishing. . . .

Not all is despair, however. Research is providing some answers. New technologies are being devised to solve the special solid waste problem erected by the used car that nobody wants any more.

[These new methods include] . . . development of the electric steel furnace, . . . shredding units, . . . giant hammer mills, . . . a giant auto-eater . . . which . . . [can] reduce a full-size car to pellets of "cleaned" steel, . . . a somewhat analogous monster known as a "frag-menter," . . . [a] new high-speed Japanese auto salvager, . . . operating [by] crushing and cooking . . . cars, . . . [new] car crushers (portable and stationary), new shearing equipment, and new shredders. . . .

—Small, *Third Pollution*, pp. 81, 84–86.

The automobile accounts for more than half of the deaths in the 15- to 24-year-old age bracket, as compared to about 10% for heart disease and cancer combined.

—"The Price of Automobiles," *JAMA* (August 31, 1970), p. 1419.

An American doctor of 1900 announced that the horseless carriage, by replacing horses, would also drive the flies off the streets. "Thus a serious channel of infection will be done away with and many lives spared. The horseless carriage will greatly reduce the death rate in cities."

—Antony Jay and David Frost, *The English* (New York: Stein & Day, 1968).

4

Water Pollution

＊

Today, the average American uses about 150 gallons of water daily. Not all of this is really necessary, as you would soon find out if you had to pump it by hand and tote it back to the house the way our ancestors did.

—Ottinger, *What Every Woman Should Know*, p. 37.

On a per capita basis, poor tropical countries use less than 5 gallons [of water] per day. Small rural communities in England use perhaps 20 gallons per day. Similar United States communities use twice as much. Large commercial towns in England use about 50 gallons a day while the average in the United States for such towns is closer to 200 gallons. The highest per capita water consumption of any city in the world is that of Beverly Hills, California (over 500 gallons per person per day), where in an arid climate immense lawns are kept sprinkled the year round and countless swimming pools are filled and refilled.

—Donald E. Carr, *Death of the Sweet Waters*, (New York: Norton, 1966), p. 69.

In 1965, 270 billion gallons of water per day were used in the United States. By the year 2020, 1,370 billion gallons—more than 5 times as much—will be needed. Hydrologists estimate that the total usable supply from precipitation is only 700 billion gallons per day. This means that the difference will have to be met by recycling water from industries and municipalities for reuse.

In each reuse cycle the chemical concentrations increase.

—*Environmental Health Problems*, p. 25.

. . . [One] of the richest water resources is the aquifer, the vast underground supply that is largely replenished by rain seeping into the ground—or would be, except that more and more of the rain water doesn't get into the ground. Instead, it is lost as runoff into the sewers. How much water do we lose this way? The major U. S. highways alone cost us well over 355 *billion* gallons each year and the highways planned for construction over the next 30 years will rob us of an additional 1.5 *trillion* gallons. When you add up the billions and billions of gallons that are lost as a result of runoff from other streets and roads and sidewalks, it's no wonder that people in areas like Long Island are now discovering that groundwater supplies are dwindling dangerously.

—Ottinger, What Every Woman Should Know, p. 38.

[Glenn Seaborg, Atomic Energy Commission:] By 1980, we will be producing enough sewage and other water-borne wastes to consume, in dry weather, all the oxygen in all 22 river systems in the United States, while the need for fresh water will have almost doubled.

—Environmental Health Problems, p. 45.

Approximately 8 million Americans drink water with a bacteriological content that exceeds the limits of the United States Public Health Service Drinking Water Standards.

—Environmental Health Problems, p. 24.

Millions more Americans are served by water supplies that are under inadequate surveillance, contain serious defects, or are operated by poorly qualified personnel.

Presently, nearly half of our 20,000 community water supply systems contain defects that are serious enough to place them in a potentially unsafe status if the defects are not corrected.

—Environmental Health Problems, p. 24.

The evidence is that water-borne communicable disease from bacteriological contamination is still a problem in the United States. Example:
    —In Riverside and Madera, California, 20,000 people were made

ill in 1965 in water-borne disease outbreaks. Several deaths were charged to these episodes.

—*Environmental Health Problems*, p. 25.

A reliable estimate has been made that a minimum of 40,000 cases of water-borne illness occur each year.

—*Environmental Health Problems*, p. 26.

According to the latest data of the pollution control agency, only some 140 million Americans of the nation's 200 million people are served by any kind of sewer system. The sewage of nearly 7 per cent of those 140 million, including many right in New York City, is discharged "raw," or untreated. With only about 85 million of the nation's people does sewage get the "secondary," or two-stage, treatment now considered minimal.

Yet many states have resisted Federal intervention. Iowa contended last year [1969] that it was unconstitutional. Colorado's Gov. John A. Love is on record as saying it would be "traitorous" for states to submit to Federally prescribed water quality standards.

—Gladwin Hill, "Purification of Nation's Waters Expected to be Long and Costly," *The New York Times* (March 17, 1970), p. 29.

Experts estimate that less than 40 per cent of our municipal sewage gets adequate treatment—and that is a very optimistic estimate. As a result, we are dumping at least 15.8 trillion gallons of filth into our water each day and the burden increases faster than we are building treatment facilities to cope with it.

—Ottinger, *What Every Woman Should Know*, pp. 43–44.

Current projections . . . are generally premised on providing only two-stage treatment for sewage—precipitation of gross solids and neutralizing of most of the other pollutants by biological or chemical action. But this leaves some stubborn residual substances, notably nitrogen and phosphorous—natural fertilizers that propagate undesirable plant growths in waterways, disrupting their entire ecology.

The belief is growing that the only ultimate solution is widespread "tertiary" or three-stage treatment, which will remove practically all adulterants and leave clean, if slightly saline, water.

This costs twice as much as two-stage treatment (including amortization of plant costs), but is already being applied on a small scale in a number of places. . . . [This kind of treatment is seen] as essential, for instance, in rehabilitation of the Potomac, now overburdened with inadequately treated District of Columbia sewage.

—Hill, "Purification of Nation's Waters Expected to be Long and Costly," *The New York Times* (March 17, 1970), p. 29.

. . . [Another] problem is urban storm-water runoff. In most communities it goes down the same pipe as the sewage, and often is nearly as dirty. But the volume at the time of a downpour is more than any sewage plant can handle. So sewage plants customarily "blow the switch," diverting large amounts of both storm water and sewage toward waterways untreated.

The only solution is to separate sewage and storm-water conduits and somehow handle storm water by itself.

—Hill, "Purification of Nation's Waters Expected to be Long and Costly," *The New York Times* (March 17, 1970), p. 29.

Present-day problems that must be met by sewage treatment plants can be summed up in the eight types of pollutants affecting our waters. The eight general categories are: common sewage and other oxygen-demanding wastes; disease-causing agents; plant nutrients; synthetic organic chemicals; inorganic chemicals and other mineral substances; sediment; radioactive substances; and heat.

—*A Primer on Waste Water Treatment*, Federal Water Pollution Control Administration, U.S. Department of the Interior (Washington, D.C., 1969), Publication No. 1969 0–335–309, p. 10.

To complicate matters, most of our wastes are a mixture of the eight types of pollution, making the problems of treatment and control that much more difficult.

—*A Primer on Waste Water Treatment*, p. 13.

The Committee on Pollution of the National Academy of Sciences has compiled a long list of pollutants which enter the watercourses of the U.S., all of which have at least laboratory proof of their potential hazard in both freshwater and marine environments. Outside of the laboratory, only the acute and more direct effects of contaminants upon the health and welfare of man are well documented and described.

> —Jay Chamblin, "Rumblings from the Deep," *Science News*, Vol. 96, No. 11 (September 13, 1969), p. 214.

There are some 12,000 different toxic chemical compounds in industrial use today. Over 500 new chemicals are developed each year.

Many of them enter and contaminate both surface waters—rivers, streams, lakes, oceans—and ground waters—water within the earth that supplies wells and springs.

> —*Environmental Health Problems*, p. 25.

Chemical contamination has been implicated in several diseases. There are indications that certain organic chemicals are cancer producers.

> —*Environmental Health Problems*, p. 26.

Some chemicals occur naturally in water but most are introduced by the waste waters from our expanding industries and municipalities. Most conventional treatment processes, originally designed to produce water that is bacteriologically safe, *do not appreciably change* the chemical characteristics of the water.

> —*Environmental Health Problems*, p. 24.

While it has always been assumed that community water systems could transform even tainted water supplies into something harmless and potable, that assurance is wearing thin.

"Our treatment plants," says Dr. C. C. Johnson, head of the Department of Health, Education and Welfare's consumer protection division, "are not designed for, nor are they prepared to take the chemical onslaught now coming from our streams."

> —Hill, "Purification of Nation's Waters Expected to be Long and Costly," *The New York Times* (March 17, 1970), p. 29.

A new fright in water contamination was aroused by a discovery in 1960 of Dr. Shih Lu Chang of the Robert A. Taft Sanitary Engineering Center at Cincinnati. This was the fact that otherwise pure water from various American rivers contains microscopic worms called nematodes, which can carry pathogenic bacteria and viruses. These nematodes are able to withstand chlorination and other severe treatment and act as protectors of the microorganisms attached to them. Thus a nematode can slip through a whole water purification system, carrying in its stomach, so to speak, the undigested bacteria. The worms are known to breed in sewage-disposal plants.

Nematode infestation has been found in treated drinking water from the Mississippi, the Colorado River in California, from the Missouri, from the Potomac in Maryland, the Columbia, the Chattahoochee in Georgia, the Delaware in Pennsylvania, the Detroit River, the Rio Grande in Texas, the Merrimack in New Hampshire and Massachusetts, the Niagara in New York, and the Tennessee River.

—Carr, *Death of the Sweet Waters,* pp. 47–48.

A Federal General Accounting Office study last year concluded that despite the expenditure of $1.2-billion in Federal grants and $4.2-billion by localities for new sewage treatment facilities, there had not been improvement in the quality of the nation's waterways.

"In the last 10 years," says David D. Dominick, the . . . Commissioner of the Federal Water Pollution Control Administration, "the quality of the nation's water has probably degenerated."

—Hill, "Purification of Nation's Waters Expected to be Long and Costly," *The New York Times* (March 17, 1970), p. 29.

. . . [Though] President Nixon prescribes an increased dose of technology to cure pollution, his medicine may well have side effects. Consider his $10 billion plan to build new primary and secondary minicipal water-treatment plants. While such plants do make water cleaner, they also have two serious faults. Unlike more expensive tertiary treatment plants, they do not exterminate man-killing viruses, like those that cause infectious hepatitis. They also convert organic waste into inorganic compounds, especially nitrates and phosphates. When these are pumped into rivers and lakes, they fertilize aquatic plants, which flourish and then die. Most of the dissolved oxygen in the water is used up when they decompose. As a result, lakes "die" in the sense that they become devoid of oxygen, bereft of fish, choked by weeds.

—"Fighting to Save the Earth from Man," *Time* (February 2, 1970), p. 62.

Elimination of phosphates from detergents would not solve the eutrophication problem. There are too many other sources of these chemicals in municipal, industrial, and agricultural wastes. The treatment of municipal wastes is of particular importance in minimizing eutrophication. If these were managed properly, phosphates arising from human wastes and from detergents would be simultaneously eliminated. Effective treatment also would attenuate the flow of organic matter into lakes.

—Philip H. Abelson, "Excessive Emotion about Detergents" (editorial), *Science*, Vol. 169, No. 3950 (September 11, 1970), p. 1033.

The current drive to eliminate phosphates from detergents could lead to the replacement of safe chemicals by potentially hazardous ones.

—Abelson, "Excessive Emotion about Detergents," *Science* (September 11, 1970), p. 1033.

The Federal Government succeeded last week in undoing several years of public education on the harm that detergents do to the nation's waters. In an action as unnecessary as it was sudden and confusing, four of its top health and environmental officials urged a return to phosphate detergents on the ground that alternative cleansers were worse. . . .

—"Whitewash for Phosphates" (editorial), *The New York Times* (September 22, 1971), p. 46.

WASHINGTON, Sept. 15—In a major reversal of environmental policy, Federal officials told American housewives today to return to the use of phosphate detergents.

The health and environment officials said that detergents containing phosphates, which they acknowledged cause ecological damage, were a lesser evil than cleaners that contain either caustic soda or the chemical NTA, both of which are harmful to humans.

69

In effect, the officials said that the modern chemical technology that invented the detergents that produce cleaner clothing had also led to the pollution of waterways and had raised hazards to the public health of humans, some potentially serious.

To retain extra-clean clothing, the officials said . . . , the public must pay a price ecologically, at least for a while.

—Richard D. Lyons, "Return to Detergents With Phosphates Urged by Government in Shift of Policy," *The New York Times* (September 16, 1971), p. 1.

The Environmental Protection Agency suggests now that the solution must lie in the building of special sewage treatment facilities, or the adaptation of existing plants, with a view to ridding effluents of all harmful phosphates, not just those from detergents. . . . The trouble is that governments move at the pace of a leisurely snail; by the time essential equipment is installed, untold damage may be done. . . .

—"Whitewash for Phosphates," (editorial), *The New York Times* (September 22, 1971), p. 46.

Detergent makers and phosphate suppliers welcomed the Government's statement . . . [on September 15, 1971] backing the use of phosphates in detergents, although some companies expressed disappointment over the continued ban on nitrilotriacetic acid, or NTA, as a substitute ingredient to build the power of the detergents.

—Gerd Wilcke, "Detergent Companies Hail U.S. Step on Phosphates," *The New York Times* (September 16, 1971), p. 37.

. . . [NTA] is even more effective than phosphates as a cleaner. . . .

Last year, however, some scientists . . . warned that NTA seemed to be causing birth defects when fed to laboratory animals.

Questions have also been raised about the potential cancer-causing effects of NTA. . . .

. . . [Government officials have] pointed out that the very property that makes NTA a good ingredient in a detergent—its ability to neutralize minerals—could also make it an environment hazard, perhaps even worse than phosphates.

Technically, NTA has the ability to combine with heavy metals such as mercury. The resulting combination is then deposited in the ground, where it enters the food chain and is concentrated by plants that are eaten by animals that are eaten by people.

Because heavy metals such as mercury and cadmium are known to cause diseases, especially harmful effects to the brain, scientists have questioned the increasing use of NTA.

—Lyons, "Return to Detergents with Phosphates Urged by Government in Shift of Policy," *The New York Times* (September 16, 1971), p. 37.

When the Federal Government cautioned against the use of NTA a year ago, many detergent makers started marketing products that contained neither NTA nor phosphates. In other formulations the amount of phosphates in the detergent was extremely low.

Most of these new preparations contained alkalies, such as caustic soda, which are one of the main ingredients of soap. But the alkaline preparations may also be hazardous.

Dr. [Charles C.] Edwards [the head of the Food and Drug Administration] said, for example, that the caustic agents might damage the eyes, nose and throat. He noted that there were 3,900 poisonings in the United States last year from cleaning products such as these and said that the risk of accident was especially high among children.

—Lyons, "Return to Detergents With Phosphates Urged by Government in Shift of Policy," *The New York Times* (September 16, 1971), p. 37.

Less harm would be done for the time being if housewives continued, with reasonable care, to use so-called caustic sodas, especially in combination with regular soap. A nation that suffers the lethal automobile and allows handguns is not likely to be overwhelmed by the presence of washing sodas in the home—along with a dozen other potentially risky substances such as drain cleansers, dangerous drugs or even kitchen matches. Time, moreover, gives promise of producing really harmless detergents, several of which are reported to be well on the way.

A holding pattern of this sort, rather than the implausible course the Government has chosen, would allow a continuing effort to save the nation's waters without causing more than a minimal risk to health. . . .

—"Whitewash for Phosphates" (editorial), *The New York Times* (September 22, 1971), p. 46.

71

. . . [It] is estimated that, because of phosphates, from both detergents and human wastes, Lake Erie has aged 15,000 years in the last half-century.

> —Lyons, "Return to Detergents With Phosphates Urged by Government in Shift of Policy," *The New York Times* (September 16, 1971), p. 37.

Lake Erie, in scientists' estimation, is an ecological disaster area. Lake Michigan is heavily contaminated in some areas. Even the clarity of Lake Superior is threatened.

> —Hill, "Purification of Nation's Waters Expected to be Long and Costly," *The New York Times* (March 17, 1970), p. 29.

The cost of cleaning up Lake Michigan alone has been expertly estimated as high as $10-billion. The ultimate prospective cost of cleaning all the nation's waterways is out of sight, somewhere beyond $100-billion.

> —Hill, "Purification of Nation's Waters Expected to be Long and Costly," *The New York Times* (March 17, 1970), p. 29.

. . . [The] Federal Water Quality Administration of the U.S. Department of the Interior is gambling the biggest single project grant in its history on the conviction that a workable substitute for indiscriminate dumping into the lakes is at hand. FWQA is committed to spend $2-million on the opening phase of a research project intended to demonstrate that sewage and factory effluent presently being poured into Lake Michigan can be diverted to fertilize barren land in Michigan. If all projections for the scheme prove out, this new waste disposal system will pay for itself and net a profit, perhaps even stimulate the economy of Michigan by building up an agro-industrial complex of respectable size.

> —John R. Scheaffer, "Reviving the Great Lakes," *Saturday Review* (November 7, 1970), p. 62.

The Great Lakes Basin is made up of glacial outwash plains. Large stretches of well-drained soil suitable for irrigation lie within reach of urban centers but beyond commuting zones and thus are susceptible to purchase at unexploited farmland prices. If we take the Muskegon

[Michigan] irrigation tract as a model, simple mathematics tells us that a billion gallons of waste water per day (that is the flow rate of Chicago's sewage disposal system, the largest in the country) can be disposed of on 260,000 acres of land. A preliminary survey of the major metropolitan areas of the United States suggests that all of them could be served in this same manner by using marginal lands equivalent to no more than 2 per cent of the acreage on which fifty-nine principal crops were harvested in 1968.

—Scheaffer, "Reviving the Great Lakes," *Saturday Review* (November 7, 1970), p. 65.

In Michigan, . . . a 500-acre land and water complex will present the management of waste water from a modern waste disposal plant so that nutrients and contaminants are handled as resources capable of being converted into useful products. . . .

Several interlocking biological recycling systems, designed as an alternative to discharging treated wastes into streams, have been developed by the Institute of Water Research (IWR) at Michigan State University. . . .

These biological systems . . . include a conventional waste treatment plant, an aquatic system of shallow lakes, and a land system of laboratories, wooded areas, and open field plots. The complex will handle 2 million gallons of secondary treated liquid waste per day (equivalent to sewage from 30,000 to 40,000 people). These land and water systems will be combined with a community recreation project to provide complete recycling of the waste water. . . .

Rooted aquatic plants will be grown in these . . . lakes to maximize the removal of phosphates and nitrates from the secondary effluent. . . .

. . . [Each] lake will support underwater plant life that will be harvested three or four times a year. . . .

What the harvested crop will be used for remains a question. One answer is to feed it to livestock. . . . Another possibility is the extraction of proteins from this material for feeding the increasing human population.

—Carol E. Knapp, "Recycling Sewage Biologically," *Environmental Science and Technology*, Vol. 5, No. 2 (February 1971), pp. 112–13.

OTTAWA, April 15—President Nixon and Prime Minister . . . Trudeau signed a joint treaty today to begin the large-scale job of cleaning up the Great Lakes, the world's largest reservoir of fresh water.

Under the agreement, the United States plans to spend $2.7 billion to $3-billion over five years in Federal, state, local and private funds, and the Canadians will spend about one-seventh that amount.

> —Robert B. Semple, "Great Lakes Pact Signed in Ottawa by Nixon, Trudeau," *The New York Times* (April 16, 1972), p. 1.

A Ralph Nader task force has come up with a harsh and apparently accurate assessment of the government's efforts at cleaning up water pollution. After 15 years (the National Water Pollution Control Act was passed in 1956), seven laws, and the expenditure of $3.5 billion, says the report [*Water Wasteland*], the level of filth has not been reduced in a single major body of water. Industry's share of pollution —now four to five times as much as that from domestic sources— continues to rise. The country's ranchers, loggers, and farmers, who form the agricultural pollution sector, continue to be the "worst polluters in the entire nation."

> —Constance Holden, "Nader Group Sees 'Water Wasteland'," *Science*, Vol. 172, No. 3982 (April 30, 1971), p. 455.

The Hudson River's lower reaches are filthy. Major rivers like the Ohio, the Mississippi and the Missouri are still heavily polluted. The Detroit River, the Cuyahoga at Cleveland, and the Houston ship canal are essentially industrial sewers.

> —Hill, "Purification of Nation's Waters Expected to be Long and Costly," *The New York Times* (March 17, 1970), p. 29.

. . . [The] Cuyahoga River in Ohio is so overrun with volatile industrial discharges that last summer [1969] it caught fire and burned two railroad trestles.

> —"The Ravaged Environment," *Newsweek* (January 26, 1970), p. 36.

The Houston Ship Canal, a 57-mile-long waterway that links the southwest port to Galveston Bay and the Gulf of Mexico, has so little natural flushing that, as one official put it, "virtually everything that keeps the channel wet is industrial effluent."

—"The Ravaged Environment," *Newsweek* (January 26, 1970), p. 37f.

About half of the 500 square miles of shellfish beds in Galveston Bay, adjacent to the Houston area, are classified as polluted and unfit for harvesting. The industrial waste situation is aggravated by discharges of inadequately treated municipal sewage from Houston and its environs.

—Gladwin Hill, "Texas Pollution Spurs Action by U.S.," *The New York Times* (January 19, 1970), p. 33.

One giant [kraft-paper mill] on the Coosa River, which runs through Georgia and Alabama, pours into the stream wastes equivalent in oxygen demand to untreated sewage from a city of 200,000 persons.

—Carr, *Death of the Sweet Waters*, p. 150.

LONDON — A distinguished panel of experts warned Tuesday [February 23, 1971] that environmental pollution has reached the stage where it threatens the quality of life in Britain.

This was one of the many conclusions set forth in the first report issued by an independent Royal Commission on Environmental Pollution. . . .

The commission raised these major points . . . :

—The state of some British rivers is depressing. Too many of them are now polluted to the point where recycling or reuse of the water is impossible.

—Britain's estuaries and coastal waters are increasingly treated as an open drain and dumping ground. . . .

—Richard Reston, "British Experts Warn Pollution Perils Life," *Los Angeles Times* (February 24, 1971), p. 26.

Near Marseille, a pair of big aluminum refineries each day discharge 6,000 tons of a red sediment into the Mediterranean. Though 80% of it funnels into a deep submarine trench, the remainder settles elsewhere on the bottom. "The problem," says [Alain] Bombard [a famed marine biologist], "is that this waste, though not toxic in itself, blankets and kills all living things. Moreover, this is an area where it is essential to have living water to purify the sewage of Marseille."

> —"Fighting to Save the Earth from Man," *Time* (February 2, 1970), p. 61.

Another growing problem is "thermal" pollution of waterways by heat from industrial cooling water, particularly power plants. Some fish species are blighted by as little as a four-degree chronic alteration of their accustomed milieu.

Thermal pollution will worsen as atomic power plants, which produce more waste heat, replace conventional fossil-fueled plants.

> —Hill, "Purification of Nation's Waters Expected to be Long and Costly," *The New York Times* (March 17, 1970), p. 29.

Insufficiently treated human wastes are another source of damage to marine ecosystems. Lifeless zones have been created in the marine environment; there have been heavy kills of fish and other organisms. Shellfish have been found to contain hepatitis, polio virus, and other pathogens. . . .

> —Philip H. Abelson, "Marine Pollution," *Science*, Vol. 171, No. 3966 (January 8, 1971), p. 21.

Along with radiation, critics of the reactor program are alarmed about the effects of thermal pollution on marine life. The problem is that nuclear plants use cool water from rivers and bays, then return it hot. All steam-generated plants require cooling water—as do many other basic industries—but reactors can use as much as 35% more water because they use heat less efficiently than plants fueled by coal or oil. Heat decreases the dissolved oxygen content in the water, makes existing pollutants more toxic, disturbs the reproduction cycle of fish and spurs the growth of noxious blue-green algae.

> —"The Peaceful Atom: Friend or Foe," *Time* (January 19, 1970), p. 43.

. . . [Too] much algal life deprives fish of the oxygen they need and eventually kills them or forces them away. Without the natural control exerted by the fish population, the algae undergo a phenomenon known as "algal bloom." They proliferate in such quantity that they completely dominate the aquatic environment and the water becomes syrupy and clogged. Not only is this bad for the waterway and the fish, it's also very bad for people. Algal bloom produces noxious gases so unpleasant that people can't live near them and so corrosive that they have actually been known to eat the paint off houses.

—Ottinger, *What Every Woman Should Know*, p. 35.

Heat reduces the water's oxygen content. The water has to be cooled and *aerated* before it is returned [by the power plant].

—Ottinger, p. 35.

Scientists estimate that by 1980, the plants producing the nation's electric power will require some two hundred billion gallons of water per day, nearly all of it for cooling purposes. As noted in the January —February 1968 issue of the *Sport Fishing Institute Bulletin*, "This compares to an annual nationwide runoff totalling 1,200 billion gallons per day. In other words, a quantity of coolant equivalent to one-sixth of the total amount of available fresh water will be necessary for cooling the steam-electric power-producing plants. . . ."

—Richard Curtis and Elizabeth Hogan, *Perils of the Peaceful Atom* (New York: Doubleday, 1969), p. 145.

The ecology of any given area—the relationship of each plant or animal to every other organism in the environment—is always an extremely complex and delicately balanced system. An apparently insignificant change in one branch of that system can have astonishingly significant effects on another, and indeed on the interrelationships of *all* parts. The eradication of a large portion of a river's fish population, then, is not merely pathetic in terms of the fish and the humans who directly depend on them for food and sport; it may be tragic in the many unpredictably dire consequences suffered by all life in the environment.

—Curtis and Hogan, *Perils of the Peaceful Atom*, p. 143.

. . . [Heat] has a profound effect upon the composition of water itself. Warm water can hold less oxygen dissolved in solution than cooler water. Since fish must obtain needed oxygen from water by means of their gills, a drop in the oxygen content of water leads to suffocation and death. When a body of water already contains toxicants of other kinds near the maximum allowable tolerances—as is the case with an increasing number of America's waterways—even a relatively small rise in temperature can have disastrous consequences.

> —Curtis and Hogan, *Perils of the Peaceful Atom*, p. 143.

. . . [Salmon] along with other fish of the salmon family such as trout, are particularly sensitive to temperature changes. The Pacific Northwest's Columbia River Basin is a major salmon spawning ground, but it is also the site of considerable nuclear reactor activity. Scientists now calculate that this activity will raise the temperature of the river to 85 degrees Fahrenheit, a full *five degrees above the maximum temperature tolerable by salmon even for a few hours*. Even a temperature of anything approaching 85 degrees, then, could result in nothing less than the complete extirpation of the river's salmon population, sending one of the most valuable natural resources on the North American continent to the same fate as the extinct, or all but extinct, bison, sperm whale, alligator, and passenger pigeon.

> —Curtis and Hogan, *Perils of the Peaceful Atom*, pp. 143–44.

. . . [A] rise in temperature of only a few degrees can enable formerly dormant fungi and parasitic organisms to flourish in water. Such has recently been observed in the Columbia River, due essentially to the discharges of the Hanford [nuclear] reactors. The net effect has been the growth of a deadly, but hitherto dormant, bacterial fish disease, columnaris. The disease has taken a heavy toll of salmon swimming upstream toward their spawning grounds.

> —Curtis and Hogan, *Perils of the Peaceful Atom*, p. 144.

Even if . . . fish are not slaughtered outright by excessive heat or columnaris, or even if excessive heat can be controlled, the fish population is nevertheless endangered by even moderate rises in water temperature. Cyclical changes in water temperature are vital to the reproductive processes of such fish as bass, trout, salmon, and walleyes. Unless they experience the natural rhythm of seasonal variations, their reproductive mechanisms will be disoriented, disrupted, or destroyed. Furthermore, a relatively slight upward change in water temperature can prove fatal to fish eggs and small fry, so that the attainment of the desired spawning grounds—an incredibly difficult struggle for many varieties of fish under the best of circumstances—does not guarantee the hatching of eggs or the development of the fry.

—Curtis and Hogan, *Perils of the Peaceful Atom*, p. 144.

... [*Virtually*] *every large fresh-water system in our country is earmarked for nuclear plant cooling purposes!*

—Curtis and Hogan, *Perils of the Peaceful Atom*, p. 144.

There *is* one way to combat thermal pollution, and that is by means of "cooling towers" designed to lower the temperature of water emerging from reactors before it is returned to its source. Since these cost millions of dollars, however, utilities seek to avoid adding them to their facilities. The AEC [Atomic Energy Commission] does not require them as standard equipment.

—Curtis and Hogan, *Perils of the Peaceful Atom*, p. 145.

On Lake Michigan alone, seven nuclear power plants, several with capabilities larger than any in the history of power generation, are scheduled to be in operation by the mid-1970s. Together with the output around the lake of existing plants fueled by coal and oil, the higher volume of expelled heated water will raise the temperature of all of Lake Michigan by several degrees in the next few decades.

... Yet, incredibly, not one of the plants is installing cooling towers to reduce the environmental impact of the heated water on this vital segment of the Great Lakes chain—a major resource of international importance.

—Gaylord A. Nelson (U.S. Senator), "Our Polluted Planet," *The Progressive*, Vol. 33, No. 11 (November 1969), p. 14.

We must know in advance that wiping out forests destroys the soil, ruins lakes and streams, even affects the climate and causes some agricultural crops to die. We must know that digging a canal to the ocean can admit sea lampreys and wipe out our lake trout fishery. We must know that phosphates in detergents will fill our lakes with fast growing algae.

If we are to . . . save the natural resources of this land to sustain ourselves and future generations . . . [then] we must begin at once to develop the governmental programs and institutions which will accomplish that life or death goal.

—Nelson, "A Congressional View of the Problem," *Proceedings*, p. 453.

. . . [Scientists] and commercial fishermen recognize three ways in which shellfish can become contaminated, depending on the kind of pollution present:

•Biological contamination of shellfish by municipal waste is well known: From inadequately treated sewage, human pathogenic bacteria, and perhaps viruses, frequently render this important food unfit for consumption.

•Paralytic shellfish poisoning of humans is caused by another pollution problem: Excess plant nutrients and even well-treated sewage can enhance the growth of certain marine organisms capable of producing toxic substances that become concentrated in the tissues of shellfish. Consumption of such contaminated mollusks is often fatal.

•And shellfish can become toxic when they accumulate excess environmental supplies of zinc or copper in concentrations several million times the amounts of these metals present in the water around them.

—Chamblin, "Rumblings from the Deep," *Science News* (September 13, 1969), p. 214.

One [pollution source] is agricultural wastes, ranging from manure to fertilizer, which some officials have suggested may be responsible for as much contamination as municipal and industrial wastes. Little has been done about it because it is hard to get at.

—Hill, "Purification of Nation's Waters Expected to be Long and Costly," *The New York Times* (March 17, 1970), p. 29.

80

[Report from the Secretary of Agriculture to the White House, issued in January 1969:] "Animal wastes are a concern in the abatement of water, air, and soil pollution. They are associated with eutrophication of lakes, fish kills, nitrate contamination of soil and aquifers, off flavors, annoying odors and dust, dissemination of agents infectious to animals and man, depreciation of recreational values of rural land and streams, and reproduction of insect pests."

—Small, *Third Pollution*, p. 48.

. . . [In] truly efficient packing houses the waste from slaughtering and butchering is minimal. But it is not negligible. There are wastes—and hazards. The daily kill-day discharges of waste water from meat-packing operations average more than 15 million gallons and contain at least 70 dry tons of suspended solids in addition to 25 to 40 dry tons of animal fats. Most of the solids are scraps from the floor. (The protein content in these scraps and the wasted blood and scraps from these [slaughtering and butchering] operations would be enough to feed several large cities.)

—Small, *Third Pollution*, p. 50.

The canning industry is a large water user and the farmers who sell their vegetables or fruit to the canneries are now large pesticide users. It thus takes 50 gallons of water to wash a case of canned fruit or vegetables where it took half that much twenty years ago. The pesticide winds up in the river.

—Carr, *Death of the Sweet Waters*, p. 148.

One of the major water pollution problems is the silt and debris that washes into lakes, rivers and streams when natural cover is stripped from the ground in preparation for construction. Through impoundments and other means—from the time the ground is broken until the project is completed and the surface again stabilized—this kind of pollution *can* be prevented.

—*What You Can Do about Water Pollution*, Federal Water Pollution Control Administration, U.S. Department of the Interior (Washington, D.C., 1967), Publication No. 0–265–805.

In general, private industry is united to a man against federal regulation of water pollution. They prefer state control, if any. As it is now, each state has its own set of standards for water cleanliness, most of them very tolerant. . . . For many years, the difference in water cleanliness standards between states has given industrialists a powerful club which they have not hesitated to use. They can threaten to move the plant downriver where the requirements are not so tough. Or they can threaten to move from a Northern state, grown more persnickety, to some Southern state, where one can dump anything short of straight cyanide into a stream.

—Carr, *Death of the Sweet Waters*, p. 145.

In 1965, the voters of New York [State] were called upon to approve a $1 billion Pure Waters bond issue which, according to the promise of the moment, was going to clean up the waters of the state by 1970. A few years later, the deadline was 1972. By 1970, the deadline had receded into a vague "after 1974" and New York's water was still getting dirtier.

—Ottinger, *What Every Woman Should Know*, p. 45.

The federal effort has been no better [than state efforts]. The Clean Waters Restoration Act of 1965, passed with so much hope and promise, has turned out to be a disaster. The major financing plan . . . is so unrealistic as to be fanciful.

—Ottinger, *What Every Woman Should Know*, pp. 45–46.

The main problem [in federal water pollution control efforts], as the [Ralph Nader] task force perceives it, is in the "weakness of basic federal laws regulating pollution." . . . The federal law, says the report [Water Wasteland], leaves too much responsibility to the states, which, subject to local political pressures, have less stringent codes on pollution and are often even less willing to take action than the federal government is.

The task force feels that the WQO [Water Quality Office] will have to give up the idea of trying to solve problems in a chummy "partnership" atmosphere with polluters and state officials. Instead, the

WQO should adopt an "adversary" stance that will not tolerate endless compromises, empty assurances, and the repeated pushing back of cleanup deadlines.

> —Holden, "Nader Group Sees 'Water Wasteland'," *Science* (April 30, 1971), p. 455.

Efforts to implement the water quality standards face total collapse because the Federal aid commitment is not being met. In 1968, $450 million in Federal aid was authorized by Congress, but only $203 million was appropriated. For 1969, $700 million was authorized, but less than one-third that figure was appropriated.

> —Nelson, "Our Polluted Planet," *The Progressive* (November 1969), p. 15.

Several years ago, a survey reported in the *Harvard Business Review* indicated that this [effective abatement and restoration of our water supplies] might cost us as much as $4 billion a year over the next 30 years. This is considerably less than half what we spend on tobacco annually; in fact, the taxes we collect on tobacco alone each year could pay for the entire cleanup job.

> —Ottinger, *What Every Woman Should Know*, p. 44.

A cost estimate and study was made to get a clearer picture of how much it will cost to meet all of the pollution control requirements for municipalities, industry, and other entities.

The estimate is: $26 billion to $29 billion will be needed to collect and adequately treat municipal and industrial wastes discharged into the nation's waterways in the 5-year period beginning July 1, 1968. This would cost each American approximately 26 dollars per year—or 50¢ per week.

> —*Showdown*, Federal Water Pollution Control Administration, U.S. Department of the Interior (Washington, D.C., 1968), Publication No. 0–320–380, p. 22.

. . . [Most] forms of industrial pollution affecting navigable waterways (almost anything is a navigable waterway and if it isn't, it certainly pours into a navigable waterway) are illegal already—and have been for over 70 years. The so-called Refuse Act of 1899 requires the U.S. Army

Corps of Engineers to halt every type of pollution *except* sewage. It sets fines of up to $2,500 and rewards you with half the fine if you provide the information leading to the conviction of a polluter. Unfortunately the present United States Attorney General, John G. Mitchell, has announced that he doesn't intend to enforce the law, so the only way you can make the law work is to bring action in a federal court to require him to act.

I strongly recommend this course of action. My husband [then Congressman Richard Ottinger] brought such an action to halt the Penn Central Railroad's pollution of the Hudson River with oil from its switching yards in Harmon. The railroad was fined $4,000 and the $2,000 bounty was turned over to the Hudson River Fishermen's Association to finance similar prosecutions.

—Ottinger, *What Every Woman Should Know*, pp. 47–48.

One of the most useful antipollution tools is the newly rediscovered Refuse Act of 1899, which bans most dumping into navigable waters without a permit from the Army Corps of Engineers. It specifically encourages citizen complaints, even entitling informants to one-half of any resulting fine set by a court.

Do-it-yourself kits on this law can be obtained from the conservation and natural resources subcommittee of the House of Representatives' Committee on Government Operations (Rayburn House Office Building, Washington, D.C. 20515) or Rep. Edward I. Koch (D) of New York (Longworth House Office Building, Washington, D.C., 20515).

Support for such citizen watchdogging comes directly from the nation's new antipollution chief, William D. Ruckelshaus, administrator of the Environmental Protection Agency: "I am heartily in favor of responsible citizen court actions against polluters—of citizen pressure against government at every level, including the federal government and my own agency."

—Peter C. Stuart, "Pollution: What You Can Do," *The Christian Science Monitor* (February 18, 1971), p. 9.

Ironically, pleasure boats as well as commercial vessels are one source of water pollution. Wastes from one boat may seem of little or no consequence, but wastes from many boats contribute significantly to the total water pollution problem.

—*What You Can Do about Water Pollution.*

As a garbage disposal method, dumping at sea has been largely discontinued because much of the material is washed ashore. Nevertheless, ocean dumping of refuse such as chemicals and oil refinery wastes is on the upswing, though pressure is building against it, too.

—Edward Gross, *Digging Out from Under, Science News* (September 27, 1969), p. 279.

The Federal and state governments are among the biggest polluters of coastal waters surrounding the U.S. Earlier this year [1969], during a Congressional investigation into the military's plan to dispose of surplus poison gas in the Atlantic, a high-ranking Defense Department witness testified that the military had always regarded the ocean as a kind of "Davy Jones Locker . . . where things could be put and forgotten *(Science News:* 5/24, p. 499)." And in an effort to circumvent pollution of rivers and estuaries, coastal cities are planning to build pipelines in which millions of gallons of industrial waste and municipal sludge can be sluiced directly into ocean waters beyond the continental shelves.

—Chamblin, "Rumblings from the Deep," *Science News* (September 13, 1969), p. 214.

Oil is crucial to everyday life. The U.S. demand alone is 588 million gallons a *day* and rising. Much of it has to be shipped over water: last year [1969] a billion metric tons of oil were transported in 3,800 hulls. In the process, a million tons a year are spilled, leaked or deliberately flushed into the sea. Still more oil goes directly into the water from offshore wells, 7,500 of which now ring the U.S.

—"The Dirty Dilemma of Oil Spills," *Life,* Vol. 68, No. 8 (March 6, 1970), p. 29.

. . . [Global oil] spillages have reached the point where the entire world ocean is affected.

Petroleum constituents, some suspected of causing cancer, are entering the oceanic food chain . . . and eventually could reach dining room tables. Thus, the world faces the possibility of losing the seas as a food source. . . .

This warning has been issued by Dr. Max Blumer, . . . senior scientist in the chemistry department of the Woods Hole Oceanographic Institution in Massachusetts. . . .

Annual world oil production is about 1,800 million metric tons, he said, of which at least 60 percent travels the seas. The total spillage, from leaks, accidents, flushing of bilges and tanks is, he estimates, about a million tons.

This, however, he believes to be a conservative estimate and it does not include production accidents, such as the recent leakage in Santa Barbara Channel, or industrial dumping into rivers and harbors that flow to the sea. The grand total, therefore, "is likely to be 10 to 100 times higher," Dr. Blumer said.

—Walter Sullivan, "Oil Called Peril to Food Supply in Sea," *The New York Times* (January 16, 1970), p. 18.

With the advent of supertankers—aptly nicknamed "oilbergs"—the danger increases that 300,00 [metric] tons or more may be dumped in a single mishap. Yet the vast majority of the 950 spills recorded by the U.S. last year [1969] are small, the result of minor equipment breakdowns and seemingly insignificant human error. In the aggregate, they do most of the damage. In fact, two thirds of all spillage occurs during routine pumping and transfer operations in port.

—"The Dirty Dilemma of Oil Spills," *Life* (March 6, 1970), p. 29.

In World War II 16,000-ton tankers were standard. Today 300,000-ton behemoths ply the sea, and larger ships are planned. As the *Torrey Canyon* dramatically demonstrated in 1967, one ship can cause a major calamity. In the past five years 94 tankers have foundered; two collisions occur every week. Then there is the risk of dangerous pollution from offshore oil wells. Last spring [1968] a presidential panel investigating the Santa Barbara Channel blowout concluded that the U.S. faces one major oil spill every year after 1980.

—"The Black Tide," *Time* (December 26, 1969), p. 29.

(Original Department of the Interior plans for the Santa Barbara Channel resulted in the leasing of 71 tracts, each tract capable of containing one or more . . . platforms, or comparable subsurface or bottom installations—each platform capable of drilling and servicing 60 wells. The potential total is thus over 4,000 offshore wells. In the past, according to Interior Department statistics, a blowout rate of 2.5 per thousand wells has held true. Over the next few years, if Government and industry persist in their plans for a forest of oil installation in the channel, Santa Barbara can anticipate perhaps 10 repetitions of the Jan. 28 blowout.)

—Ross Macdonald and Robert Easton, "Santa Barbarans Cite An 11th Commandment: 'Thou Shalt Not Abuse the Earth'," *The New York Times Magazine* (October 12, 1969), p. 33.

As with everything else concerning the [Santa Barbara Channel oil] spill, there were and are differences of opinion about the amount of oil spilled. Union Oil's initially quoted estimate of 5,000 barrels a day was later withdrawn, and lowered to 500 barrels a day. A scientist with General Research Corporation, Alan A. Allen, who inspected the channel every day from the air, estimated the minimum flow at 5,000 barrels a day, or over 2,000,000 gallons in the 10½ days before the well was plugged.

—Macdonald and Easton, "Santa Barbarans Cite An 11th Commandment," *The New York Times Magazine* (October 12, 1969), p. 143.

Oil blowouts are much more common than is generally realized. During 1968 alone, wild-well expert [Red] Adair was called in to control 40 blowouts, worldwide, 11 of which were offshore. When the Adair company was brought in on the Santa Barbara [oil] spill, one of the employees reported that "blowouts have become so common in the offshore fields of Louisiana that they scarcely rate notice in the newspapers."

—Macdonald and Easton, "Santa Barbarans Cite An 11th Commandment," *The New York Times Magazine* (October 12, 1969), p. 144.

. . . [The] detergents used to disperse oil slicks [on water] do more damage to marine life than the oil itself.

—"The Ravaged Environment," *Newsweek* (January 26, 1970), p. 32.

Pearl Harbor has a peculiar and sad oil-pollution problem. Petroleum fuel oil still oozes slowly up from the American warships sunk on December 7, 1941. An oil slick still forms above the USS *Arizona* Monument.

—Carr, *Death of the Sweet Waters*, p. 152.

. . . [A] beach on Barbados Island in the Antilles is fouled with tar and oil, although ships rarely pass. It is believed that the scum has been blown from afar by trade winds.

—Sullivan, "Oil Called Peril to Food Supply in Sea," *The New York Times* (January 16, 1970), p. 18.

Thor Heyerdahl, who has just crossed the Atlantic in the papyrus [boat] Ra II, reports that the vast ocean has become so polluted in places that his crew was reluctant to wash in it. He observed that "at least a continuous stretch of 1,400 miles of the open Atlantic is polluted by floating lumps of solidified asphalt-like oil." . . .

—"Trouble on Oily Waters" (editorial), *The New York Times* (July 19, 1970), The Week in Review section, p. 12.

Thor Heyerdahl, navigating the mid-Atlantic . . ., discovered plastic bottles, oily blobs and other detritus of civilization adrift on huge patches of ocean far from the nearest ship or shore.

—"The Ravaged Environment," *Newsweek* (January 26, 1970), p. 31.

. . .Ra II's oily passage offers grim evidence that there is no time to lose. If Milton's "illimitable ocean" can no longer wash away man's ills, it is obviously time mankind began to clean up its own mess.

—"Trouble on Oily Waters" (editorial), *The New York Times* (July 19, 1970), The Week in Review section, p. 12.

The potential implications of the opening up of Alaska's North Slope could keep teams of ecologists busy for years. Whether some logical order can be imposed on the development remains to be seen. What for instance would happen if a future giant oil tanker split up on the ice? "We are concerned," says Dr. Lamont Cole of Cornell University, "because these Arctic ecosystems are very fragile and can take decades or even centuries to recover from some man-imposed disaster. For instance, in warm climates an oil spill might degrade quickly, but oil up there could last a good many years."

—"Northwest Passage," *Science News,* vol. 96, no. 13 (September 27, 1969), p. 266.

Right now some ecologists are worried about the possible effect on the Eskimo of the great oil race on Alaska's remote North Slope. Oil spills in the ever-frozen sea, they fear, would be trapped in the narrow space between water and ice, killing first the plankton, then the fish and mollusks that feed on the plankton, then the polar bears, walrus, seals and whales that feed off sea life, and finally threatening the Eskimos who live off these animals.

—"The Ravaged Environment," *Newsweek* (January 26, 1970), p. 36.

Dramatic oil spills in coastal waters capture the public's concern by killing countless marine creatures and sea birds. But more pernicious is the long-term effect of chronic pollution from tankers flushing their storage compartments at sea. That, along with other everyday mishaps, adds up to 284 million gallons of spilled oil every year—about ten times the amount that oozed from the *Torrey Canyon,* and enough to coat a beach 20 ft. wide with a half-inch layer of oil for 8,633 miles. Scientists are increasingly worried that this oil could be poisonous to ocean plankton, a key source of photosynthesis that produces most of the earth's oxygen.

—"The Black Tide," *Time* (December 26, 1969), p. 29.

If the oil is killing the life along the coral heads, what must it be doing to the phytoplankton at sea which provide 70% of the oxygen we breathe?

—A. B. C. Whipple, "An Ugly New Footprint in the Sand," *Life,* Vol. 68, No. 10 (March 20, 1970), p. 20B.

It is the economic profit to be found in the sea that attracts and brings closer the threat of cataclysm which Dr. Paul Ehrlich, a noted ecologist, projected recently. He predicted that unless current trends are reversed, the oceans could end as a significant source of life in ten years with the end of man coming a short time later.

—Nelson, "Our Polluted Planet," *The Progressive* (November 1969), p. 16.

GENEVA, Oct. 25—A noted Swiss marine scientist estimated today that at the current rate of pollution there would be no life in the world's oceans in 25 years. He said that the shallow Baltic Sea, which has no tides, would be the first to die, and that the Adriatic and the Mediterranean, which also have no tides to carry away pollution, would be next.

Dr. Jacques Piccard, the scientist, who has been appointed adviser to the United Nations Conference on the Environment, to be held in Stockholm next June, said at a news conference that he hoped the conference would be able to provide practical means of averting these dangers.

He warned, however, that the remedies would be costly. The motorist already pays more for lead-free gasoline, he said. Although it is possible to manufacture paper without discharging mercury into streams, he said, it is more expensive. Governments will have to pay part of the cost.

—"Swiss Scientist Estimates Seas Will Die in 25 Years," *The New York Times* (October 26, 1971), p. 5.

5

Solid Wastes Pollution

Americans today use 50 per cent of all the raw materials grown, mined, pumped, or otherwise produced anywhere in the world. . . . We, in this country, represent less than six per cent of the world's total population, but we use half of the planet's natural wealth. In practical terms, how long can this go on?

Even more serious is what we do with what we use. We often speak of ourselves as "consumers." We are not consumers, we are users and wasters.

—Ottinger, *What Every Woman Should Know*, pp. 16–17.

In 70 years of life, the average American uses 26 million gallons of water, 21,000 gallons of gasoline, 10,000 lbs. of meat, 28,000 lbs. of milk and cream, as well as $8,000 worth of school buildings, $6,000 of clothing and $7,000 of furniture.

—"Fighting to Save the Earth from Man," *Time* (February 2, 1970), p. 59.

We throw away 3.5 billion tons of solid wastes each year.
—360 million tons are household, municipal and industrial wastes.
—2 billion tons are agricultural wastes.
—1.1 billion tons are mineral wastes.

—*Environmental Health Problems*, p. 4.

Solid wastes collected by public and private organizations amount to 190 million tons per year—or 5.3 pounds per person per day.

Estimates vary slightly, but because of the expected continuing increase in population and the trend for each individual to produce more trash, by 1980 the amount *collected* will probably be over 340 million tons per year or 8 pounds per person per day. The total refuse generated in 1980 may be more than 370 million tons.

—*Environmental Health Problems*, p. 4.

. . . [The] trash we will generate between now [1970] and 1980 would build a four-lane highway ten feet thick from here to the moon—and there would be enough left over to build some unsavory secondary roads at the other end.

—Ottinger, *What Every Woman Needs to Know*, p. 49.

Each day, urban communities across the United States produce more than 800 million pounds of solid wastes. By 1980, that figure is expected to be three times higher.

—Small, *Third Pollution*, p. 24.

Each of California's 18.5 million residents throws away 20 lbs. of solid wastes per day—an amount that in a year would make a wall 100 ft. wide by 30 ft. high stretching from Oregon to Mexico.

—"Fighting to Save the Earth from Man," *Time* (February 2, 1970), p. 60.

At present the total national expenditure for handling and disposing of municipal, commercial, and industrial solid wastes is more than $4.5 billion a year.

In spite of this impressive expenditure, most systems of solid waste disposal are inefficient.

—*Environmental Health Problems*, pp. 4, 18.

Of the $3 billion a year spent on handling municipal solid wastes alone (a conservative estimate), more than $2.5 billion goes for collection. It costs New York City an average of $26 per ton to collect refuse and transport it to an incineration facility.

—Small, *Third Pollution*, p. 40.

94

The result of massive production is massive filth. Every year, Americans junk seven million cars, 100 million tires, 20 million tons of paper, 28 billion bottles, 48 billion cans. Just to collect the garbage costs $2.8 billion a year.

—"Fighting to Save the Earth from Man," *Time* (February 2, 1970), p. 59.

The household garbage can . . . contains from 40 to 60 per cent paper in the form of newsprint, food wrappings, and other paper trash, 10 per cent throwaway bottles (and, in this affluent society, some returnables), 5 per cent plastic containers, 8 per cent assorted tin cans (including those dangerous packed-under-pressure spray cans . . .), and a few old bones, half a dozen kids' toys, 10 to 20 per cent grass clippings and leaves, a sack of vacuum cleaner dust, an old fluorescent bulb, occasionally a dead pet, and a few dozen other nondescript items that must once have had some value.

Further complicating municipal refuse disposal are today's industrial wastes, ranging from the disposable uniforms, linen, and syringes from the local hospital to radioactive material from the nearby nuclear power plant.

—Small, *Third Pollution*, p. 24.

This is still the Stone Age of waste handling: we deal with our trash the way the caveman did. We burn it, or bury it, or move away from it. (We are less mobile than the caveman. He just moved to another cave when the situation became intolerable. We move our trash to someone else's cave, but the result is the same.)

—Ottinger, *What Every Woman Should Know*, p. 54.

Solid waste experts are concerned about the great imbalance in cost between collection and disposal.

—Anton J. Muhich, then chief of systems and operations planning for the solid waste program of the Department of Health, Education, and Welfare, suggested in 1968 that the split exists because "as a nation, we have tended to emphasize collection services and have virtually ignored proper disposal practices."

—Small, *Third Pollution*, pp. 40–41.

Today, Americans are spending $4.5 billion a year for refuse collection and disposal services—domestic and industrial—a sum that is exceeded only by expenditures for schools, roads, and national defense. Yet the number of dollars spent on collection far outstrips the dollars spent on disposal—even though a startling 12 per cent of the U.S. residential population receives no formalized collection service.

—Small, *Third Pollution,* p. 49.

The deplorable condition of most of the solid waste disposal systems in the United States was brought out in a national survey, which showed that only 6 percent of landfill operations could be classified as sanitary landfills.

In a sanitary landfill operation, solid waste is buried in the ground and covered with a thin layer of soil at the end of each day to keep out insects and rats.

If only 6 percent are sanitary landfills then the remaining 94 percent consist of open burning dumps that add to air pollution or contaminate ground water and contribute to water pollution or do both.

—*Environmental Health Problems,* p. 17.

Mishandling of solid wastes is costlier than the use of good refuse disposal methods in many ways. The economic losses in medical bills; fire and rodent damage; air and water pollution; use of makeshift insect sprays, traps, and poisons; exterminators' fees; depreciated property values; and other hidden costs of dirty cities are staggering.

—Small, *Third Pollution,* p. 40.

Solid wastes have been associated with at least 22 human diseases.

Dumps, alleyway garbage heaps, and other places of garbage accumulation are excellent breeding grounds for disease carrying animals.

—*Environmental Health Problems,* p. 18.

It must be emphasized that the improper methods of disposing of refuse provide potential health hazards such as the harborage of rats,

96

breeding of flies and mosquitoes, and polluting [of] streams and ground waters, as well as contributing to air pollution.

—Charles Kurker, "Reducing Emissions from Refuse Disposal," *Journal of the Air Pollution Control Association*, Vol. 19, No. 2 (February 1969), p. 70.

An ever-increasing number of communities are turning to incineration to solve their solid-waste disposal problems. A recent study by the New York State Office of Local Government revealed the following relationship between population and method of disposal:

Sanitary landfills: 60 municipalities totaling 892,000 people

Incinerators and related fills: 66 municipalities totaling 12,200,000 people

Open dumps or private disposal: 1,420 municipalities totaling 3,659,000 people

Although this suggests that the larger municipalities utilize incineration, smaller ones will be turning to it as available fill land disappears.

—Melvin A. Benarde, *Our Precarious Habitat* (New York: Norton, 1970), pp. 163–65.

In order to conserve dumping space, refuse [in open dumps] is periodically set afire deliberately. Burning can be a solution for combustible refuse. However, it increases the load of particulate matter (smoke) and volatile chemicals in the already overburdened air and thus, of course, contributes to air pollution. Burning dumps are a major contribution to air pollution in most large cities.

—Benarde, *Our Precarious Habitat*, p. 155.

Communities are running out of places to dump their refuse, and are destroying irreplaceable resources in the frantic effort to stay ahead of the flood. A prime example is San Francisco Bay, a dumping site for years, which is now filling up to the point where conservationists fear it may one day disappear.

—Gross, "Digging Out from Under," *Science News* (September 27, 1969), p. 278.

The average American today throws away twice as much as his father did. If present trends continue, each of our children will soon be throwing away twice as much refuse as each of us.

—Ryan, "A Congressional View of the Problem," *Proceedings,* p. 343.

Logically, one solution [to the growing trash problem] would be to bury the trash in a sanitary landfill rather than dump. . . .

But . . . [the sanitary landfill] too has drawbacks, stemming largely from packaging materials of paper and plastics that do not readily compact, thereby shortening the life span of a landfill and reducing its effectiveness. Rapidly biodegradable materials would be a blessing here, but the current trend in packaging is away from them.

The landfill also does not eliminate the problems of ground water and surface water pollution and adds the problem of hazardous methane buildup and dust. And as population increases, space for landfills will be harder to get and more expensive.

—Gross, "Digging Out from Under," *Science News* (September 27, 1969), pp. 278–79.

[Sanitary landfills] . . . usually require about one acre per ten thousand people per year. Therefore, it is necessary for a community to set aside large tracts of land. In the face of the increasing demand for living space, the two needs come into conflict. . . . When refuse is buried and covered, chemical changes take place as a result of microbial activity. . . .

In a controlled, properly designed landfill, the energy released by the chemical changes . . . is so great that there is a precipitous rise in internal temperature . . . well above the temperature needed to kill the heat-sensitive pathogens. This offers a fair degree of assurance that the fill is not a health hazard. . . .

. . . With the growth of urban areas and the mass migrations to the suburbs, . . . filled land has been developed . . . for home sites. Two problems have resulted:

1. In too many instances, the settling of fill has caused houses to develop large cracks. . . .

2. In 1966, First, Viles, and Levin reported on the danger of toxic gases and explosive hazards in buildings erected on landfills. . . .

Perhaps a better solution would be to set these lands aside for much-needed parks and playgrounds.

One of the major uses of landfill is for the reclamation of otherwise unusable land, particularly marsh. However, the loss of marsh areas, which may serve as recreational sites and sources of fish, may not be completely desirable. . . . In Long Island, New York between 1954 and 1959, over 13 percent of the wetlands were destroyed by landfill projects.

—Benarde, *Our Precarious Habitat*, pp. 157–62.

Unquestionably, the [trash disposal] plans will have to be different for different types of situations. . . . Recognizing these differences, there is still one disposal method that has tremendous potential for all areas over the short run: high-heat incineration. The new high-heat incinerators operate at 3000 degrees and consume any product you are likely to find in trash except firebrick and soil. They reduce trash volume by 94 to 96 per cent. If all our trash today were processed this way, we would have only 10 to 16 million tons of residue to deal with in place of the 270 million tons that face us now. Furthermore, the residue is harmless and potentially useful. It is a clean "frit" like heavy sand which can be used in building bricks, as a covering for fireproof shingles or in construction. Because the system operates at such high heat, it produces practically no air pollution. What it does produce can readily be handled by existing abatement devices. Working on a truly regional basis, there is no reason why this clean heat can't be put to another use as well: the generation of power.

—Ottinger, *What Every Woman Should Know*, p. 55–56.

A national survey showed that about 200 of the 300 incinerators in the nation burning municipal waste lack adequate air pollution control equipment.

The figures clearly demonstrate the direct relationship between solid waste mismanagement and air pollution.

—*Environmental Health Problems*, p. 18.

The most important step is to reorganize our system for handling trash. It is largely a political problem and one where you and I can make our political muscle felt, if we try. Today most of our waste disposal operations are handled by the smallest possible political unit, such as the town or village. If a larger unit gets involved, such as a township or a county, it is usually just to provide and maintain a dump or incinerator. . . .

The really promising new developments in trash handling are very expensive and become economical only when they are constructed and operated so as to handle a large volume. But . . . [how] can a community afford the expense of a new multi-million dollar incinerator and the pollution control equipment necessary to make it safe?

—Ottinger, *What Every Woman Should Know*, pp. 54–55.

If and when some newly authorized federal funds . . . are appropriated, then state officials, sanitary engineers, and their solid waste consultants will begin to pay close scrutiny to a refuse recycling plant that literally mines today's solid wastes and makes a profit for the state or municipality over and above the disposal costs.

—Stanton S. Miller, "A Solid Waste Recovery System for all Municipalities," *Environmental Science and Technology*, Vol. 5, No. 2 (February 1971), p. 109.

The Department of the Interior's Bureau of Mines has always considered waste products and scrap generated by the mineral and metals industry and the consuming public as potential resources. . . .

It is not inconceivable that the present-day mine tailing dumps, municipal landfills, and junk car graveyards may be looked upon in the future as "man-made mines" for minerals whose natural ores have been depleted or remain in deposits that can be mined only at greater cost than required for recycling waste.

—Charles B. Kenahan, "Solid Waste—Resources out of Place," *Environmental Science and Technology*, Vol. 5, No. 7 (July 1971), pp. 595, 600.

Last year [1970], a New Jersey law put garbage collection and disposal under the aegis of the state's Public Utilities Commission (PUC). By doing so, New Jersey became the first state to attempt to solve its solid waste problem by treating garbage handling as a regulated public utility. . . . [Scientific Incineration Devices (SID)] has asked the New Jersey PUC for a nonexclusive franchise to operate disposal facilities in the state's 10 most populous counties. . . .

. . . The area has a population of about 5.3 million people and produces almost 12,000 tons of garbage daily. . . .

. . . The company plans to use high temperature incineration to dispose of the refuse at selected sites. . . .

. . . SID has operated a prototype 300 ton/day disposal facility at Wanaque, N.J., for more than a year with "excellent" results, according to . . . [its president]. Although the Wanaque incinerator is remarkable for its apparent lack of "gee-whiz" technology, the process that's used appears to be solid and reliable.

. . . Combustion temperatures between 1500–2000° F assure complete combustion (without auxiliary fuel) and avoid formation of NO_x [nitrogen oxides], which occurs at high temperatures.

. . . [The design of the incinerator is such that], SID says, . . . a clean, white steam plume is virtually all that escapes to the atmosphere.

Water used . . . is recirculated. . . . Additional water, as needed, is taken from wells.

[It is claimed] . . . that the Wanaque facility is the only incinerator currently operating in New Jersey in compliance with the state's air pollution regulations. . . . Although the Wanaque facility is not necessarily identical to those that would be installed in the proposed 10-county franchise area, the centers would operate with similar, proved equipment.

The cost of refuse disposal, if the franchise is granted, is pegged at about $6.50 per ton. As recycling industries develop, that price would drop. . . .

—H. Martin Mallin Jr., "Utility Concept of Solid Waste Handling Makes Gains," *Environmental Science and Technology*, Vol. 5, No. 9 (September 1971), pp. 752–53.

Today's mechanized trash sorters can divide solid waste material into four or five categories. Now a team headed by MIT's Dr. David G. Wilson is developing a computerized sorter that could separate half or more of a city's refuse into 50 or more reusable groups. A pilot plant, which should be starting up about now, will first sort trash into large (the size of a soda bottle or bigger) and small. Then large chunks will be whirled on turntables past a variety of sensors. These will perform analyses and report to a computer, which will identify the chunk and direct it into an appropriate chute. Unidentifiable trash and small chunks go to a pulverizer and then to separation by density.

—Arthur Fisher, "Science Newsfront," *Popular Science* (October 1971), p. 46.

A cousin to the sanitary landfill is composting, in which organic waste material is used as a soil conditioner. Unfortunately, no great agricultural market has opened for the method, mainly because of the economic difficulty of separating metal, plastic and glass from organic matter, and competition from commercial fertilizers.

—Gross, "Digging Out from Under," *Science News* (September 27, 1969), p. 279.

Separation of the various components [of garbage] at the home has been tried, and is still in practice here and there. To separate putrescible matter from non-putrescible by the use of two garbage cans is not beyond the mental capacity of the average housewife. Some cities have even required three cans.

But the practice has been unpopular with housewives, and no one blames them greatly. The regulations are difficult to enforce, and so chiselers have their chance. The conscientious housewife feels put upon.

—Stewart, *Not as Rich as You Think*, p. 92.

Grinding, flotation, and other methods can separate the organic material that is subject to decay. Either as added to the sewage or treated alone it can be considered a resource.

—Stewart, *Not as Rich as You Think*, p. 92.

A number of schemes have been advanced to get valuable urban solid wastes back into the soil. Solids removed as sludges from domestic waste waters, which in part represent the spent topsoils carried to the cities on fresh vegetables, can be incinerated to kill any micro-organisms and then trucked to farms for spreader application. . . . Pennsylvania State University is piping sewage effluent directly into fields to

102

use as irrigation water, leaving the residue of solids right in the water. (Elsewhere, agricultural wastes themselves are being recycled. Cheese whey is being sprayed on Wisconsin crop lands. Some Oregon farmers are spraying hog manure onto their grain, hay, and pasture fields with no reported pollution effects.)

—Small, *Third Pollution*, p. 56.

Composting is one of the oldest methods of disposing of solid wastes known to man. For centuries, farmers have been spreading human and animal waste and vegetable waste on the fields, returning organic matter to the soil. But modern practices and public health considerations have militated against organic fertilizers. As a consequence, composting has never really achieved wide popularity in the United States, despite its great value under properly controlled conditions.

—Small, *Third Pollution*, pp. 95–96.

Although urban waste disposal and pollution problems are getting much heavier attention in the United States at present, farming and forestry produce far more waste and contamination than do municipalities. The volume of wastes from livestock and poultry production alone is estimated at 1.7 billion tons annually. . . .

. . . Cattle are no longer herded directly from the field to the railhead for shipment to the city markets. Giant feedlots have sprung up around the major cities where cattle are held three to five months for fattening. . . . Since single feedlots often contain more than 10,000 cattle, the accumulation of several inches of manure in the feedlot is not unusual.

. . . Much of the waste is washed from the feedlots into the nearby streams, or stacked in huge piles around the pens. . . .

. . . [Some] human health problems . . . stem from diseases in animals that can be transmitted to people. Animal dung is a well-known breeding ground for flies and other insects. . . . [The] increasing concentrations of animal wastes around the major cities are causing consternation among biologists and public health officials. . . .

. . . [Many] animal diseases are caused by pests growing in animal wastes. Today, a virus or bacterial infection could spread rapidly across

103

the giant feedlots and stockyards of the nation, infecting hundreds of thousands of animals before it could be brought under control.

—Small, *Third Pollution*, pp. 43, 47–49.

. . . [The] farmers in the 1970's generally ignore the value of organic fertilizer. The cost of labor and equipment for picking it up and spreading it on the fields is high. Anyway, they argue, the natural materials would have to be supplemented with chemicals and minerals missing from natural products. Thus, in addition to the great loss of valuable material, mountains of animal wastes overload barnyards. Lagoons and streams run full with the drainage from the farmlot and pasture.

The President's Science Advisory Committee, in a special section of its report "Restoring the Quality of Our Environment," pointed out that groundwater pollution arising from the disposal of livestock and poultry wastes may be evidenced in undesirable changes in taste, odor, and color of the water. Moreover, when manure treatment or storage areas are improperly located, the nitrate levels in immediately adjacent water supplies may become disturbingly high.

—Small, *Third Pollution*, p. 46.

For every ton of tomatoes harvested by machines, three tons of waste products are left in the field.

—Small, *Third Pollution*, p. 51.

More than half of the approximately 240,000 acres of rice stubble in eight California counties is burned annually, producing a heavy smoke haze for miles. Nearly one-third of the 900,000 acres of grass grown for seed each year is burned as a sanitation measure, emitting about 50,000 tons of ash and carbon into the atmosphere. Sugarcane and orchard wastes are also burned in large quantities throughout the United States. In one California county in 1960, an estimated 41,000 tons of orchard wastes were burned.

—Small, *Third Pollution*, p. 51.

Some 18,000 industrial establishments now process farm products for food. In processing crops into food and fiber there inevitably are losses of organic and inorganic matter. . . . Recently published data indicate that the pollution potential of these wastes is equivalent to that produced by a population of more than 168 million people.

—Small, *Third Pollution*, p. 51.

Fires in U.S. forests—about 150,000 of them a year—have been estimated to release 160 cubic miles of smoke into the atmosphere annually, along with 34 million tons of particulates and 338,000 tons of hydrocarbons, both of which contribute significantly to the total air pollution of the country. Some 5 to 7 million acres of forests are lost to fires each year, at a cost reaching over $1 billion. And what is well known is that poor solid waste management in the industry is primarily to blame: forest fires fed by logging wastes are more than seven times as large, on the average, as those in timbered-off areas from which such wastes have been removed.

—Small, *Third Pollution*, p. 53.

As the population mounts, unspoiled land becomes an increasingly precious resource. And unlike the air and water, land has no internal currents to dilute its pollutants; soil, once polluted, stays that way long after the source of the pollution is removed.

—"The Ravaged Environment," *Newsweek* (January 26, 1970), pp. 38–39.

Almost all of the world's well-watered, fertile farmland is already in use. Yet each year, especially in industrialized nations, millions of acres of this land are taken out of cultivation for use as industrial sites, roads, parking lots, etc. Deforestation, damning of rivers, one-crop farming, uncontrolled use of pesticides and defoliants, strip-mining and other short-sighted or unproductive practices have contributed to an ecological imbalance that has already had catastrophic effects in some areas and over a long term may adversely affect the productivity of large sections of the world.

—The Menton Statement.

105

As the key producers, green plants alone have the power to harness the sun's energy and combine it with elements from air, water and rocks into living tissue—the vegetation that sustains animals, which in turn add their wastes and corpses to natural decay. It is nature's efficient reuse of the decay that builds productive topsoil. Yet such is the delicacy of the process that it takes 500 years to create one inch of good topsoil.

—"Fighting to Save the Earth from Man," *Time* (February 2, 1970), p. 57.

Every year, Greater Los Angeles' growth consumes 70 sq. mi. of open land. Not only is prime farm land taken out of production, but it is also developed in an inefficient way; the term "slurb" was coined in California to describe sleazy, sprawling subdivisions. By planning ahead, much land can be preserved, with houses and services concentrated between green belts. But Californians, like all Americans, have a record of acting for their own benefit only after the damage is done.

—"Fighting to Save the Earth from Man," *Time* (February 2, 1970), p. 59.

According to the latest USDA figures, sediment produced by erosion of the land probably averages at least 4 billion tons a year. Moved by flowing water from one place to another, about one-fourth of this material—more than 1 billion tons—reaches the major streams of the United States.

—Small, *Third Pollution*, p. 54.

[TVA [Tennessee Valley Authority], the nation's biggest producer of electricity, is turning its back on one of its original objectives—to preserve the land—in order to generate vast quantities of power.

More than 80 percent of TVA's power is supplied by 11 coal-burning steam plants. Last year [1970], TVA bought 32 million tons of coal. . . . Approximately half the TVA coal was strip mined.

The U.S. Geological Survey . . . study . . . [entitled] "Influences of strip mining on the Hydrologic Environment of Parts of Beaver Creek Basin, Kentucky," . . . fully documents the appalling destruction of the land and streams. In strip-mined areas, the rains washed away

27,000 tons of earth per square mile each year, contrasted to 1,900 tons in areas where strip mining had not occurred. Minerals washed out of the earth at a rate of 1,370 tons per square mile in stripped areas, contrasted to 111 tons in nonstripped areas.

—Ken Hechler, "TVA Ravages the Land," *National Parks and Conservation Magazine*, Vol. 45, No. 7 (July 1971), pp. 15–16.

The USDA report "Control of Agriculture-related Pollution" maintains:

Soil erosion and its effects are damaging many times over. First, there is the irreparable loss of soil that usually has taken many thousands of years to form. Second, sediments not only contribute heavily to suspended-solids pollution but also add to the dissolved-solids problem. Third, sediment frequently damages the area where it comes to rest, for example, lined canals where sediment furnishes a place for aquatic and other weeds to grow.

—Small, *Third Pollution*, pp. 54–55.

The Imperial Valley [in southern California] has perhaps the richest farmland in the nation, producing five or six bumper crops a year. The valley's intense irrigation, however, is raising the level of the water table to the bottom of the irrigation trenches. Salts are pulled to the surface —and salts do not evaporate. In time, the soil becomes too saline to support normal crops.

—"Fighting to Save the Earth from Man," *Time* (February 2, 1970), pp. 59–60.

To boost crop production, nitrogen fertilizers are spread liberally on California's superb farm lands. Just as people get hooked on drugs, so the soil seems to become addicted to chemical additives and loses its ability to fix its own nitrogen. As a result, more and more fertilizer has to be used. What makes the problem doubly serious is that the nitrates eventually turn up in the water supply, where they endanger human health.

—"Fighting to Save the Earth from Man," *Time* (February 2, 1970), p. 60.

107

It would be incorrect to assume that systems analysis is useful only, or even primarily, in planning a war, studying the stock market, or streamlining a business operation. It can be used to tackle the broadest range of human problems. The Indus Plains Study in West Pakistan, for example, clearly illustrates how systems analysis can be used to combat human starvation and misery. Here the problem was to restore the productivity of one of the world's greatest river systems, the Indus River and its five tributaries, each in itself a major river, and each nourishing innumerable towns and cities. For more than a century, leaks had been appearing in the more than 10,000-mile network of canals that link the rivers and irrigate the Indus plains. The result had been an increasing elevation in the ground water table so that land that was once cultivated was becoming swampland and lakes. The increased water salinity that both damages plant roots and causes rapid evaporation was ruining about 100,000 acres a year.

A physical model representing the entire range of problems on the Indus plains could have been constructed. But it would have been far less flexible and adaptable than the computer model that was actually created, consisting of coded instructions on punched cards describing every sort of experimental approach. Without actually going to the expense and time of performing the experiments, the Indus plains computer study simulated the various ways the water table could be lowered—by drainage ditches, leak sealing in the canals, pumping out water by sinking wells, and so on. The plan eventually adopted proposed a grid of 32,000 wells covering about 25 million acres. The plan also recommended that each phase of the work should involve at least a million acres, to avoid water seepage from adjacent regions.

The full-scale engineering suggested by the computer has paid off. More than two million acres of land have thus far been recovered, an area capable of feeding four million additional people, and the water levels are falling at the predicted rate of 12 inches a year.

The Indus plains study involved a holistic approach, in which every possible contingency was allowed for. Of course, it requires continuing analysis to make every allowance for changing conditions—the effects of new methods of cultivation, fertilizers, insecticides, roads, pumping stations, human occupation, and the like.

In contrast to the Indus plains study, another project, the Aswan Dam in Egypt, shows how disastrous can be the failure to use the systems analysis approach in solving problems. The dam was built at a tremendous cost to provide more cultivable land and electricity for adjacent areas. What was not foreseen, but could have been predicted by systems analysis, was that the dam would alter the course of the tributary rivers of the Nile and change the chemical content of their water. Today, the salt content of this water has risen to dangerous levels, harmful to plants and thus worse than useless for irrigation. The quantity and variety of fish are diminishing. Simultaneously, bilharzia, the snail-borne disease, is on the increase because the traditional one-crop irrigation process has been replaced by four-crop rotation. Nutriments deposited annually by the Nile flood are severely depleted, and this is reducing the fertility of the soil. Already, the changes wrought by the dam have had unfortunate effects on the fisheries of the eastern Mediterranean.

The results of this project are likely to be ultimately catastrophic. Yet they could have been foreseen and prevented if long-range planning had been substituted for shortsighted, short-term vision. Had a systems analysis study been carried out long before the first spadeful of earth was moved, the story would have been very different. Quite probably no dam would have been built, and a massive program of population control would have been mounted in its stead. In some instances, making more land available for cultivation may be the worst thing for a nation to do. Where before there were only a small number of people living on the edge of starvation, unplanned soil recovery may cause a substantial increase in the number of people who more than ever continue to live near the edge of starvation.

—Ashley Montagu and Samuel S. Snyder, *Man and the Computer* (Philadelphia: Auerbach, 1972), pp. 139–141.

The . . . [Aswan High Dam on the upper Nile] has . . . stopped the flow of silt down the Nile, which in the past offset the natural erosion of the land from the Nile delta. As a result, downstream erosion may wash away as much productive farm land as is opened up by the new irrigation systems around Lake Nasser [behind the dam]. Without the nutrient-rich silt reaching the Mediterranean, the Egyptian sardine catch declined from 18,000 tons in 1965 to 500 tons in 1968.

—"Fighting to Save the Earth from Man," *Time* (February 2, 1970), p. 62.

. . . [An] important phase of mineral disposal lacks a name, and we may coin for it the term "counter-erosion." Everyone recognizes the bad effects of erosion, but few seem to have focused upon the problem of what becomes of the material that is eroded away.

. . . Along a few miles of highway, many tons of earth may wash away. This material . . . gets into the natural drainage. . . . It tends to throw out of adjustment the natural and long-established balance of the stream-flow. . . . If the drainage is unobstructed by lakes or dams, the material starts on a long journey toward the sea. . . . More commonly, these days the silt lodges behind a man-constructed dam, which is thus reduced in efficiency. . . .

—Stewart, *Not as Rich as You Think*, pp. 158–59.

Land spoilage is not restricted to the urban developers. More than 20,000 strip mines are cutting ugly scars across the landscape at an estimated rate of 153,000 acres annually. By 1980, according to a White House study, more than 5 million acres of America the Beautiful will have been defaced in this way. Before it passed stiff reclamation laws, the lush green state of Kentucky was gorged by strip mines to the extent of 119,000 acres. In Florida, a process described as "surface mining" in which carloads of ore and earth are scooped up from the land, has stripped some 150,000 acres.

—"The Ravaged Environment," *Newsweek* (January 26, 1970), p. 39.

The second major source of solid wastes and contamination in the United States after agriculture is mining, with its associated processing industries. More than 20 billion tons of mineral wastes have been heaped upon the United States over the past thirty years, damaging or covering 7,000 square miles of land.

—Small, *Third Pollution*, p. 58.

Much of the economy of Appalachia is dependent upon the extraction of natural products—especially coal—from the ground; in the Appalachian region, . . . unwise exploitation . . . has left thousands upon thousands of acres devastated. Erosion of the damaged land pours silt and mine acid into the streams, polluting hundreds of miles of fine waters, and mine and mine waste fires belch forth thousands of tons

110

of pollutants into the air. And the people live in poverty, proof of Theodore Roosevelt's warning: "To skin and exhaust the land instead of using it so as to increase its usefulness will result in undermining in the days of our children the very prosperity which we ought by right to hand down to them."

—Small, *Third Pollution*, pp. 59–60.

Tourists are beginning to leave Appalachia nowadays; poisonous acid from strip mines has seeped into the water table.

—"Fighting to Save the Earth from Man," *Time* (February 2, 1970), p. 59.

The President's Science Advisory Committee estimates that during 1963 some 5.6 billion tons of material were mined in the United States, of which 3.3 billion tons were waste rock or mill tailings discarded at the site of operation.

—Small, *Third Pollution*, p. 62.

. . . [The] Department of the Interior has estimated that about 2 million acres of mining-disturbed land (approximately 800,000 mined for coal and 400,000 for sand and gravel) requires some kind of reclamation program. This amounts to a strip a mile wide extending from New York to San Francisco. The task of reclamation in such an area makes a "crash program" unfeasible.

—Small, *Third Pollution*, p. 66.

Mining companies spew so many wastes over tiny East Helena, Mont. (pop. 1,490) that the lettuce [grown] there contains 120 times the maximum concentrations of lead allowed in food for interstate shipment.

—"Fighting to Save the Earth from Man," *Time* (February 2, 1970), p. 59.

Not only do Americans fail to mine efficiently the materials that they have, but they waste the materials that they do mine. Leftover materials in waste piles all over the United States would be usefully and economically reworked in less affluent countries.

—Small, *Third Pollution*, pp. 67–68.

About 100 million tons of blast furnace and open hearth slags have accumulated in the Pittsburgh area alone.

—Small, *Third Pollution*, p. 71.

Culm banks and coal waste piles are largely residual waste from processing coal. . . . When these banks are accidentally ignited—as they frequently are when trash and rubbish discarded in strip pits or near the banks are deliberately set on fire—they . . . pose a menace to public health and safety as they emit noxious gases and fumes, endanger nearby surface lands and property, and destroy valuable resources (many burning for decades).

—Small, *Third Pollution*, p. 69.

The Bureau of Solid Waste Management, formerly in the Department of Health, Education, and Welfare, but recently made a part of the new Environmental Protection Agency, has been funding studies to look at the problem of construction and demolition wastes. One study covered four cities in New Jersey—Paterson, Clifton, Passaic, and Wayne. These four communities generate 116,690 tons of construction and demolition wastes per year—or 310 tons a day. This figure is for an area with a population of about 321,000.

—Small, *Third Pollution*, p. 30.

About 80 per cent of our discard is made up of paper in one form or another. Every year we cut down 3.4 billion cubic feet of trees to make paper. But recycled paper is just as good as the original.

—Ottinger, *What Every Woman Should Know*, p. 17.

. . . New York City disposes of 350,000 tons of newsprint per year, at great cost in dollars, air pollution, and litter. . . . By processing the paper in a modern, pollution-free plant for re-use by the newspaper industry, the streets and skies of New York would benefit, the tax dollar would go further, distant streams would be less polluted by effluents from paper mills, and extensive woodland areas would be conserved.

—Eisenbud, "Environmental Protection in New York City," *Science* (November 13, 1970), p. 712.

About half of the total production of paper and paperboard in the United States is used for packaging purposes—25.2 million out of the total of 46.6 million tons in 1966, for example.

—Small, *Third Pollution*, p. 23.

. . . [The] chemical industry has polluted the housewife's food package not only through the unintended absorption of pesticide residues, but also through innumerable colorings, additives (like the cyclamates) and preservatives designed to increase food purchases and consumption. . . . The package itself, which is a sales boosting device par excellence, can be both the most polluting and dangerous feature of all. As a pièce de résistance, the chemical industry produces the non-biodegradable plastic container, which . . . if made from polyvinyl plastic, like Dow's Saran-Wrap, can be deadly in the most literal sense of the word. When Saran-Wrap is accumulated as trash and burned, it produces phosgene gas—a poison gas used in World War I and currently stockpiled by the Department of Defense. Exposure for only a short duration to 50 parts of phosgene per million parts of air will cause death. The chemical industry currently makes approximately five billion pounds of polyvinyl plastic per year. . . .

—Martin Gellen, "The Making of a Pollution-Industrial Complex," *Ramparts*, Vol. 8, No. 11 (May 1970), p. 23.

The plastics industry is running wild with new ideas for packaging. . . . The market in 1966 was for 1,804,000,000 pounds for packaging alone, about 20 per cent of the total plastics produced. By 1976, this figure will double, according to current projections.

—Small, *Third Pollution*, p. 23.

The use of aluminum in packaging had approached 1 billion pounds in 1968—a 100 per cent increase over five years!

—Small, *Third Pollution*, p. 23.

Tax money . . . might be much more profitably spent in stimulating or even subsidizing the process of recycling. During the Second World War our housewives flattened their tin cans, and put them out for collection. Housewives could do so again, a slight premium being of-fered—perhaps trading-stamps or a bingo prize. The tons of cans thus collected would be kept out of the garbage and also out of the litter. In the end, the total operation would doubtless be much cheaper. . . .

—Stewart, *Not as Rich as You Think,* p. 130.

. . . Bowie, Md., is believed to be the first [community] in the country to ban the sale of soft drinks and beer in non-returnable containers. And Dr. [Ellis L.] Yochelson, more than anyone else, is responsible. . . .

. . . [He] was asked to speak to a group of students . . . at Bowie Senior High School [on Earth Day, 1970]. . . .

"I have a natural interest in solid waste," he [later] explained, with a paleontologist's fascination for life's leftovers. "An aluminum can is going to stay around as long as a billion years. A glass bottle, for all practical purposes, forever."

He talked to the students . . . about the need for recycling containers. . . .

. . . Dr. Yochelson and schoolteacher friend Don Murphy . . . [mobilized] students to poll the community on the idea of banning one-way beverage containers . . . collect 1,400 signatures on petitions . . . distribute leaflets door to door . . . enlist support from interested groups such as the Parent-Teachers Association . . . and buttonhole each city councilman before the vote.

The result: a city ordinance prohibiting the sale of no-deposit, no-return containers for soft drinks and beer . . . under penalty of $100 a day.

Since then, a handful of communities have followed. Scores of cities and several states (including Maryland) are considering doing so. And Congress has been asked by Rep. Joseph P. Vigorito (D) of Pennsylvania to impose a nationwide ban.

—Stuart, "Pollution:What You Can Do," *The Christian Science Monitor,* February 18, 1971, p. 9.

In general . . . the economic system works against salvage and recycling of materials. When there are shortages, as during World War II, people voluntarily save everything from balls of string, wax, and tinfoil to metal scrap and newspapers. But when everything is easy to come by, few persons can be bothered to return empty pop bottles or worry about junked automobiles and the litter from packages of all sorts, worn-out tires, television sets, radios, and discarded furniture. The economic incentive is toward throwing away the vital natural resources that make up these products.

—Small, *Third Pollution*, p. 95.

. . . The law . . . might be more effectively directed, not at the individual litterbug, but at the wholesale producer of unnecessary litter, that is, at the manufacturer.

The requirement of a properly-designed and installed trash basket in every automobile would be helpful and reasonable. Most service stations now have some kind of barrel or oil-drum where rubbish can be dumped; the maintenance of such a can . . . should be obligatory. . . .

The aluminum can should be flatly outlawed. . . .

The "self-opening" can should either be outlawed or re-modeled [so that] . . . [the] tab . . . would remain attached to the can.

Bottles might well be legally standardized as to sizes and shapes, so they could be recycled more economically. . . .

. . . [The] French wine industry . . . operates on an absolute minimum of variety of bottles. Except for Champagne and Alsace, all France gets along on two shapes, two colors, and one standard size. Bottles scarcely occur as litter in France. . . . [Re-use] is made easy by standardization. . . .

—Stewart, *Not as Rich as You Think*, pp. 127–28.

. . . KAB [Keep America Beautiful] has calculated that the materials jettisoned on or along the roads in one year amount to a bulk of 18 million cubic yards. . . .

An estimated fifty million dollars is expended yearly to remove litter from only the so-called "primary highways." Even so, the highways are not clean, and often are filthy.

Even more discouraging is the cost of retrieval per item. . . . Nevada estimates that the cost of the collection of *one* item from the highway is *ten cents*. Many other estimates have run much higher.

115

We have here a kind of final *reductio ad absurdum.* Our people throw worthless objects away, and then, through taxes, pay fantastic amounts to have the worthless objects picked up.

—Stewart, *Not as Rich as You Think,* pp. 119, 129–30.

As compared with certain peoples, beyond doubt, the Americans are nothing better than slovenly. Public campgrounds in Norway or Sweden, for instance, seem immaculate in comparison with those in our national forests. . . .

—Stewart, *Not as Rich as You Think,* p. 117.

6

Radioactive Pollution

Today there are 17 nuclear plants operating on the nation's waterways and 99 more under construction or in the planning stage.

—Ottinger, *What Every Woman Should Know*, p. 32.

At the present state of the art, nuclear plants definitely are neither reliable nor clean and they are probably not as safe as their supporters claim.

—Ottinger, *What Every Woman Should Know*, p. 32.

The basic fault lies with the Atomic Energy Commission (AEC) which is charged by Congress with regulating the expansion of nuclear power but which actually has put a good deal more effort into promoting it.

—Ottinger, *What Every Woman Should Know*, p. 32.

Scientists who formulate radiation protection standards say that safety is not the only consideration. For example, the International Commission on Radiological Protection reported: "At the present time, risk [health] considerations can at best play only a very general role in specific recommendations . . . and operational and administrative convenience must of necessity be of equal importance."

—Roger Rapoport, "Catch 24,400 (or, Plutonium is my Favorite Element)," *Ramparts*, vol. 8, no. 11 (May 1970), pp. 16–21.

Do nukes [nuclear power plants] leak radioactive material? Yes. There is no dispute about that. Their emissions include strontium, cesium, iodine, krypton, and tritium. What is disputed is whether these emissions are harmful. The AEC [Atomic Energy Commission] has estab-

119

lished what it believes to be acceptable levels of radiation exposure. It maintains that present emissions represent only a small fraction of that level. There are two things wrong with this. First, nobody really knows what an acceptable level of exposure is; at best the figures are calculated guesses. Second, the claims about the degree of exposure are in some cases based on questionable data and in others are simply not borne out by the facts.

—Ottinger, *What Every Woman Should Know*, p. 33.

Uncertainty exists only as to the minimum dosage that will be harmful, either to the individual exposed or to future generations. But it has been obvious that society cannot await full scientific assessment before instituting rigorous control measures.

—Small, *Third Pollution*, p. 74.

. . . [The Atomic Energy Commission points out] that we are already subjected to considerable radiation from natural sources. They say what we get from nukes [nuclear power plants] now is only a minute fraction of what we are already getting from other sources. More critical experts point out that that is just the problem. We've achieved a fairly comfortable tolerance in relation to the amount we are getting, so why increase it? And increase it we will. Dr. [Edward] Radford [a Johns Hopkins University radiologist], quotes U.S. Public Health Service figures indicating that if nuclear power grows as expected, "we would have the maximum permissible concentrations of radioactive krypton in the world's atmosphere by the year 2060."

—Ottinger, *What Every Woman Should Know*, p. 34.

Although a Nobel Prize was awarded for research done in 1927 on the genetic effects of radiation, there is still controversy over what constitutes safe exposure to radiation. Most scientists agree that there is a 50% chance that adults exposed to 450 rems of radiation will die. [Rem is an acronym for "roentgen equivalent, man." One rem is the quantity of any radiation that will have the same biological effect on man as the exposure to one roentgen of ordinary X ray.] Below about 50 rems, no visible damage has been measured. With little empirical evidence, the

AEC [Atomic Energy Commission] has adopted 500 millirems (one millirem is one-thousandth of a rem) as the maximum radiation that the general public can be exposed to in one year. That is a very small amount. By comparison, the sun and other natural radiation sources expose the average individual to about 100 millirems each year. A single chest X ray can double the natural dose.

—"The Peaceful Atom-Friend or Foe," *Time* (January 19, 1970), p. 42.

Last month [December 1969] two scientists at the AEC's Livermore Radiation Laboratory reported that current radiation standards may be responsible for as many as 16,000 additional cases of cancer a year in the U.S. and urged that exposures be cut tenfold. Though other AEC officials rebut that finding, other federal radiation experts feel that standards should be re-examined.

—"The Peaceful Atom-Friend or Foe," *Time* (January 19, 1970), p. 42.

The fact that effects of atomic experiments and programs are often totally unexpected and discovered only after radioactivity has been introduced in quantity into the environment was brought out in "Test Fallout and Water Pollution," an article by Dr. Barry Commoner which appeared in the December 1964 issue of *Scientist and Citizen*. Dr. Commoner said: "Massive nuclear testing which began with the development of the hydrogen bomb in 1953 was well under way before most of its biological consequences were appreciated. The unanticipated tendency of world-wide fallout to deposit preferentially in the North Temperate Zone was unknown until 1956; the hazard from radioactive iodine and carbon–14 was not brought to light until 1957; the special ecological factors which amplify the fallout hazard in the Arctic were elucidated for the first time in 1960; experiments which suggest that strontium–90 may cause hereditary damage by becoming concentrated in the chromosomes were first reported in 1963."

—Curtis and Hogan, *Perils of the Peaceful Atom*, p. 149.

Some years ago, it was discovered that Eskimos were absorbing far more fallout radioactivity than people living in temperate zones, even though the distribution of fallout was believed to be just the reverse. . . . The

121

answer to this puzzle lay in the enormous concentrating ability of the Arctic food chain. The first link in this chain is the tough, scrubby lichen, which has the unusual characteristic of deriving its mineral nourishment from the air instead of from the soil. Ordinarily, dust and soil particles settling on the lichen provided it with needed minerals; when radioactive fallout joined the dust and soil, the lichen absorbed it too. These plants were and are extremely efficient collectors of fallout. They are also one of the principal foods of the caribou . . . [which] in turn are an important . . . food of Eskimos . . . [who] go on receiving, as fallout continues to drift down from the stratosphere, radiation exposures which are close to, and in some cases may exceed what are considered maximum permissible exposures. . . .

—Sheldon Novick, *The Careless Atom* (Boston:Houghton Mifflin, 1969), pp. 98–99.

There are many kinds of radioactive wastes produced by the nuclear industry. AEC licensing procedures and regulations deal with more than 900 radioisotopes of 100 elements. Wastes containing these isotopes may be in the form of gases, liquids, or solids; the environmental hazard from each similarly affects the biological organism. The volumes of low-level solid wastes now being produced for commercial burial are estimated at 1 million cubic feet for 1970, 2 million by 1975, and 3 million by 1980.

—Small, *Third Pollution*, p. 74.

. . . [The] estimate of how much radioactivity we are being exposed to is based upon some questionable assumptions. Tritium is a good example. The AEC [Atomic Energy Commission] claims that tritium, which is almost weightless, escapes quickly into the upper atmosphere where, they say, it is relatively harmless to man. A distinguished radiologist at Johns Hopkins University takes sharp issue with this simplistic view. "What happens if the wind isn't blowing up and what happens when it rains?" asks Dr. Edward Radford. "I'll tell you what happens. If the wind is blowing away from the plant, tritium goes downwind with it. If it's raining, the tritium adheres to dust particles or raindrops and settles down to earth just like the fallout from an atom bomb test."

—Ottinger, *What Every Woman Should Know*, p. 33-34.

. . . [Once] released into the atmosphere, there is no conceiveable way of retrieving radioactive gases; once entered on their winding course through the environment, radioactive isotopes are out of reach of man's control.

—Novick, *The Careless Atom*, p. 124.

. . . [Public] attention has been distracted from a threat far more insidious even than the overheating of water resources [by nuclear power plants]; that of radiological pollution of the environment.
. . . [This] error has enabled power companies to play down the importance of low-level emissions of radioactivity into air and water and rule them out as valid grounds for opposition to nuclear plants. It is imperative that this gross missapprehension be corrected.

In the first place, and foremost, is the fact that many waste radionuclides take an extrardinar[il]y long time to decay. . . .

Thus even though . . . long-lived isotopes may be widely dispersed in air or diluted in water, their radioactivity does not cease. It remains, and over a period of time accumulates.

—Curtis and Hogan, *Perils of the Peaceful Atom*, pp. 148–49.

Thousands of curies of radioactivity go down the drains and into the urban sewage treatment systems, albeit in small dosages. This lethal litter of nuclear contamination is raising the background level of radiation for the entire world.

—Small, *Third Pollution*, p. 73.

Dr. Robert Pendleton, molecular biologist and genetic biologist of the University of Utah, has stated that at Oak Ridge, Tennessee, "very small amounts of radioactive waste were dumped into . . . White Oak Lake. Fish that appeared afterward . . . were fantastic. They changed into many grotesque shapes and sizes. The most amazing thing was not the genetic mutations but the fact that some fish were found many miles downstream from the lake glowing like Christmas trees."

—Curtis and Hogan, *Perils of the Peaceful Atom*, p. 153.

Man is by no means the only creature in whom radioactive isotopes may concentrate. Indeed, the dietary needs of all vegetable and animal life dictate the intake of specific elements. Those elements, whether radioactive or not, will concentrate even in the lowest and most basic forms of life. They are then passed up food chains, chains such as grass-to-cattle-to-milk-to-man. As they progress up these chains, the concentrations increase, sometimes by hundreds of thousands of times. Norman Lansdell, in his book *The Atom and the Energy Revolution*, reports a study of the Columbia River in the western United States in which it was found that while the radioactivity of the water was relatively insignificant,

1) the radioactivity of the river plankton was 2000 times greater;

2) the radioactivity of the fish and ducks feeding on the plankton was 15,000 and 40,000 times greater respectively;

3) the radioactivity of young swallows fed on insects caught by their parents in the river was 500,000 times greater; and

4) the radioactivity of the egg yolks of water birds was more than a million times greater.

—Curtis and Hogan, *Perils of the Peaceful Atom*, p. 152.

. . . [Strontium–90] is picked up from the environment by plants and animals and is accepted physiologically as the equivalent of calcium. Among animals it is stored in the bony tissues, from which it gives off ionizing radiation. Almost all of this radiation is absorbed close to its source, with damage particularly to the growing cells of the bone marrow. It can give rise to leukemia or other forms of cancer.

—Small, *Third Pollution*, p. 74.

Cobalt 60 has a half life of over five years, strontium 90 of over twenty-seven years, and cesium 137 of over thirty years. A few [radioactive isotopes] take far, far longer [to decay]. A pound of carbon 14, could it have been placed in the tomb of Narmer, Egypt's first known pharoah, around 3200 B.C., would still have more than half its potency today. A gram of plutonium 239 buried today will have lost only half its radioactivity in the year 25,969.

—Curtis and Hogan, *Perils of the Peaceful Atom*, pp. 148–49.

Speaking before a conference on Nuclear Power and Environment held in Vermont in September 1968 . . . [Barry Commoner] told . . . of an important biological observation . . . [concerning] the radioactive isotope of iodine, iodine 131.

Iodine 131 is . . . relatively short-lived, with a half life of only about eight days. . . .

Because of its short life, I–131 contamination from nuclear explosions was for a long time neglected, Dr. Commoner pointed out. In due time it was recently realized that actually it is among the most hazardous of all fission products because iodine is concentrated in the thyroid gland, and even low concentrations of the radioactive variety would, in the process of decay, severely damage the thyroid and cause harmful biological changes, among which is thyroid cancer.

—Curtis and Hogan, *Perils of the Peaceful Atom*, pp. 149–50.

A study now being conducted by the Department of Health, Education, and Welfare illustrates how tentative our information on acceptable levels of radiation exposure is. Even in its preliminary state, the study has uncovered evidence that the human thyroid gland is at least "two to three times more sensitive to radioactive iodine than we once thought." If this is confirmed by further analysis, it will mean that the present level set by the AEC [Atomic Energy Commission] for [radioactive] iodine exposure is based on a 200 to 300 per cent error in calculating human reaction.

—Ottinger, *What Every Woman Should Know*, p. 33.

The Atomic Energy Commission (AEC) has lowered the maximum permissible radiation emission rate at the perimeters of nuclear power plant facilities to five millirems a year, a reduction by a factor of 100. (A millirem is a measure of radiation absorbed by the body.) . . . John Gofman, a harsh critic of the amount of radiation persons could allowably receive under the former AEC standards, noted that the AEC is "obviously responding sensibly to sensible pressures."

—"Spectrum," *Environment* (July–August 1971), p. 26.

In the official . . . [Atomic Energy Commission] booklet "USAEC—What It Is, What It Does," . . . it is claimed that, "The AEC has an impressive safety record. For example, since the beginning of the atomic energy program in 1942 there have been only seven deaths from nuclear causes among atomic energy workers in the United States." But U.S. Public Health Service studies show that 142 uranium miners have already died because of radiation overdoses ranging as much as 500 times over the safe level. And Charles C. Johnson, Jr., head of the U.S. Consumer Protection and Environmental Health Service, says, "Of the 6000 men who have been uranium miners, an estimated 600 to 1100 will die of lung cancer within the next 20 years because of radiation exposure on the job."

—Rapoport, "Catch 24,400," Ramparts (May 1970), pp. 18–19.

Radiation problems in the reactor industry . . . begin in the shafts of uranium mines. Uranium ore also contains radium and other radioactive substances; radium, in the process of slow decomposition, releases radon, which is a gas. When the ore is mined, radon gas and its own decomposition products accumulate in the mine shaft and pose a severe hazard to miners. . . . A study performed between 1935 and 1939 revealed that approximately half the deaths among miners were due to lung cancer, and that 80 percent of the remaining deaths were due to other lung diseases.

—Novick, The Careless Atom, pp. 130–32.

Twelve million tons of radioactive sand, the refuse of uranium mining in the Colorado River Basin, is heaped in largely untended piles in an area affecting at least seven states in the Southwest. For nearly twenty years these sands have been accumulating, being blown by the wind into neighboring communities, and being washed by the rain into the tributaries of the Colorado River and eventually into Lake Mead: a water system which provides water for drinking and irrigation to parts of California, Nevada, Utah, Wyoming, Colorado, New Mexico and Arizona.

—Novick, The Careless Atom, pp. 132–33.

AEC [Atomic Energy Commission] negligence has spread the hazards of uranium mines into homes in western mill towns, allowing more than 300,000 tons of uranium mill tailings (which emit the same radon gas that has led to high incidence of lung cancer in uranium mines) to be used as construction fill in little towns like Grand Junction, Colorado.

—Rapoport, "Catch 24,400," *Ramparts* (May 1970), p. 19.

DENVER, Sept. 26—A controversy involving nine states, Congress and the Atomic Energy Commission is coming to a head in Colorado over the health dangers of leftover radioactive sands used by builders in thousands of locations. . . .

The problem centers on a form of radioactive trash: sandy material called "tailings" that have been dumped out by uranium mills since the beginnings of the atomic age.

By 1969, an estimated total of 83 million tons of uranium mill tailings had piled up in Colorado, Utah, Wyoming, South Dakota, Arizona, New Mexico, Texas, Washington and Oregon. . . .

Although the ore-processing mills from which the tailings come were licensed and rigidly controlled by the Atomic Energy Commission, some are known to have given the tailings away free to builders who found them an excellent base and backfill material for concrete slabs, patios and basements in homes, offices, factories and public buildings.

In Colorado, an estimated total of 150,000 to 200,000 tons of tailings were given away for such uses between 1953 and 1956 from a single mill in the city of Grand Junction. . . .

The [Colorado] State Health Department, backed by the Federal Environmental Protection Agency and . . . a six-man medical advisory committee, has recommended that all tailings be removed from within 10 feet of all habitable structures. . . .

Removal was recommended last week in a . . . Federal-state steering committee on the problem. . . .

. . . The Atomic Energy Commission and the United States Public Health Service voted against the recommendation.

Such a removal program . . . could cost $20-million in Colorado alone. . . .

[The AEC] has maintained for years that the tailings are not its responsibility. [Colorado] State health officials say the commission created the problem and must pay for solving it. . . .

. . . Glen E. Keller Jr., president of the [Colorado] board of health, sharply rejected any suggestion that the matter was not one for Federal action.

"I submit that the Federal Government has exercised extreme irresponsibility in this situation," he said. . . .

. . . Dr. Martin Biles of the AEC's division of occupational safety . . . said [in a letter] that health departments in all nine uranium milling states had been warned in a letter sent March 7, 1961, that tailings were a potential health problem.

. . . [The] Colorado Department of Health . . . could find no trace of such a letter. The other eight state health departments involved were asked by the Colorado department if they could find such a letter. None found any trace of it.

—Anthony Ripley, "Radioactive Building Sand Stirs Dispute," *The New York Times* (September 27, 1971), pp. 1, 15.

Equally pressing is the problem of permanent storage for lethal radioactive wastes contained in spent reactor fuel elements. The practice now is to dissolve the fuel rods in nitric acid, then store the liquid in vats underground. Already the AEC [Atomic Energy Commission] has more than 80 million gallons of this lethal liquid (which includes wastes from weapons production) in tanks that must be constantly cooled and scrupulously maintained for hundreds of years before the radioactivity is spent. The AEC is now perfecting ways to solidify the wastes to permit storage in underground caverns. Even so, the growth of nuclear power could make future storage difficult.

—"The Peaceful Atom-Friend or Foe," *Time* (January 19, 1970), p. 43.

. . . [A 1969] report of the General Accounting Office [GAO] on the AEC's management of high level wastes [from nuclear reactors] . . . found that the AEC was storing 93 million gallons of wastes at sites near Richland, Washington; near Idaho Falls, Idaho and on the Savannah River near Aiken, South Carolina. A good deal of the liquid wastes was leaking out of its containers and escaping into the ground.

128

Most of the hot stuff, about 74 million gallons, was stored at Richland, from the Hanford works. Leaks were found in 10 of 149 underground storage tanks which did not have provision for secondary containment.

According to the GAO, 227,400 gallons of high level, radioactive, liquid waste leaked into the ground. It contained approximately 140,000 curies of cesium-137.

—Richard S. Lewis, "The Radioactive Salt Mine," *Science and Public Affairs* Bulletin of the Atomic Scientists, Vol. XXVII, No. 6 (June 1971), p. 27.

. . . [Radioactive] products such as cesium-137 and iodine-131 are accepted by organisms as substitutes for other minerals and stored in the organs and soft tissues of the body.

—Small, *Third Pollution*, pp. 74–75.

In 1968, . . . a quantity of oil that had been contaminated by plutonium [at the Rocky Flats plant of the Atomic Energy Commission (AEC)] was scooped up, placed in a drum and trucked off from Rocky Flats to the official AEC burial grounds. En route, however, the drum began to leak, contaminating over a mile of highway. The AEC's solution was to repave the road. Unfortunately, plutonium's half-life of 24,400 years is a good deal longer than the full-life of asphalt, and many years from now, when the road bed wears away, the hot plutonium will be exposed, to contaminate unborn generations.

—Rapoport, "Catch 24,400," *Ramparts* (May 1970), pp. 17–18.

Apart from the hazards of low-level radiation, there is the danger that a major reactor accident could release lethal amounts of radiation into the air.

—"The Peaceful Atom-Friend or Foe," *Time* (January 19, 1970), p. 42.

On December 12, 1952, an experiment . . . being conducted at the NRX reactor, at Chalk River, Ontario [resulted in an accident]. . . .

Due to the effective functioning of emergency procedures, no one at the plant was injured during the accident, and although many were exposed to radiation, the exposures were relatively mild. . . .

. . . Five years after Chalk River, there was another near-catas-
trophe, this time in England, at Windscale Pile No. 1, a reactor used
for military purposes. This accident was far more serious than the one
at Chalk River, and resulted not only in the total loss of the reactor,
but in the release of large amounts of radioactivity into the air. Fortunately the plant was in a sparsely populated area. . . .

. . . [The] history of . . . [these accidents] teaches the same lesson:
there will always be an element of human failure no matter how
carefully a reactor is designed; and a reactor is such a complex mechanism that very often it will behave in unexpected ways. . . .

In 1964, T. J. Thompson of the Massachusetts Institute of Technology wrote that there had been nine serious reactivity accidents since
1949 in nonmilitary installations alone. . . . Late in 1966 there was still
another serious accident, at the Enrico Fermi plant at Lagoona Beach,
Michigan; . . . this accident was potentially the most serious of all.

—Novick, *The Careless Atom*, pp. 1–11.

In 1966 the Fermi reactor [near Detroit] was disabled by an accident
that released no radiation, and it is still closed. According to a study,
if all the radioactive material contained in the Fermi plant were blown
into the air during a thermal inversion, 67,000 people could die of
radiation poisoning. Even if only 1% of the radiation were released,
there would be 210 fatalities.

—"The Peaceful Atom-Friend or Foe," *Time* (January 19, 1970), p. 42.

The accident . . . at Fermi . . . is particularly disturbing when we
examine the portion of the application to construct the Fermi reactor
called the "Hazards Summary Report," prepared by the . . . consortium
. . . which built and operates the Fermi reactor.

As is required by the AEC, the Hazards Summary Report contains a section describing the "maximum credible accident." This is an
attempt to specify an accident which is not expected to occur, but
which is the worst which the designers feel could occur. . . .

[what in fact] . . . happened was a bit worse than the "maximum
credible accident," and the results worse than foreseen by . . . [the
reactor's] designers. . . . It should be emphasized that the "maximum

credible accident" was assumed to occur at a power level fifteen times that at which the actual accident occured. In other words, the actual accident was not only "incredible," it might have been far worse.

—Novick, *The Careless Atom*, pp. 164–66.

. . . [The] fire alarm that sounded . . . on May 11, 1969 at the Atomic Energy Commission (AEC) Rocky Flats plant, 16 miles up-wind of central Denver[,]. . . signaled the latest in a series of over 200 fires . . . since the plant opened in 1953. . . .

Days later Dow Chemical Co., which operates the plant for the AEC, reported that the fire had done $45 million worth of damage and burned $20 million worth of plutonium. . . . But Dow and the AEC reassured increasingly nervous Colorado residents that no radiation had escaped. . . . AEC spokesmen declared: "No appreciable amount of plutonium escaped from the building and no offsite contamination resulted from the fire."

This was supposed to be the last word. . . .

After the May 11 fire, local scientists affiliated with the Colorado Committee for Environmental Information (CCEI) began to be skeptical of the Dow and AEC scientists. . . . [They] asked the AEC to monitor Denver area soil for possible plutonium contamination from the fire.

In August 1969, Dow-AEC refused. . . . So in the fall the CCEI's Dr. Edward Martell, a nuclear chemist . . . began conducting his own soil samples. . . . This former Pentagon specialist in nuclear weapons testing . . . announced that highly lethal plutonium oxide from Rocky Flats had definitely spread out into metropolitan Denver. . . . The contamination of Denver ranged from 10 to 200 times higher than plutonium fallout deposited by all atomic bomb testing. And it was nearly 1000 times higher than the amount plant spokesmen said was being emitted.

The AEC and Dow sprang into action to try to counter Martell's facts. . . . The [subsequent] AEC study essentially corroborated Martell's data /but/ . . . "we question his interpretation of the new information. . . . /We/ don't believe . . . /the escaped plutonium/ presents a significant health hazard to Denver." . . .

. . . Dr. Arthur R. Tamplin, an expert on the physiological effects

131

of radiation and one of the few independent AEC scientists who have dared publicly to question the organization's dangerous nuclear mythology, explains . . . ". . . If the plutonium from the May 11 fire is being redistributed as Martell suggests, then it could increase the lung cancer rate for Denver by as much as 10 per cent. This could lead to as many as 2000 additional lung cancers in Denver."

—Rapoport, "Catch 24,400," *Ramparts* (May 1970), pp. 16–18.

Despite the fact that atomic power and reactor technologies are still saturated with unknowns, these [commercial] reactors are going up in close proximity to heavy population concentrations. Some have even been proposed for location in the heart of a city. Most will be of a size never before attempted by scientists and engineers; they are, in effect, experiments. Indeed, because atomic power plants have not to date proved to be of practical economic value, they are still officially licensed by our Government under the research and development rather than the commercial clause of the Atomic Energy Act.

—Curtis and Hogan, *"Perils of the Peaceful Atom,"* p. ix.

As far back as 1957, one of the AEC's own studies suggested that a reactor built 30 miles from the nearest city could kill 3400 people, injure 43,000 and cause $7 billion damage in a bad accident.

—Rapoport, "Catch 24,400," *Ramparts* (May 1970), p. 19.

. . . [In] April of 1967, a representative of the AEC's Advisory Committee on Reactor Safeguards testified before the Joint Committee on Atomic Energy that "the ACRS believes that placing large nuclear reactors close to population centers will require considerable further improvements in safety, and that none of the large power reactors now under construction are considered suitable for location in metropolitan areas."

—Novick, *The Careless Atom*, p. 88.

At the moment, about 75 American atomic power plants are planned or under construction. It is these nuclear power plants that comprise the largest single hazard of radiation for the future. The 15 plants already built don't give much cause for optimism, since those in Michigan, New Jersey and Minneapolis are currently shut down due to malfunction.

—Rapoport, "Catch 24,400," *Ramparts* (May 1970), p. 19.

This curious bill [the Price-Anderson Act] has received surprisingly little attention in the press. It provides a straightforward federal subsidy to a multibillion dollar industry. . . . [It] effectively passes the risks of the reactor industry on to the taxpayer. Section 170e of the Atomic Energy Act is amended to read:

> The aggregate liability for a single nuclear incident (nuclear accident) . . . shall not exceed the sum of $500,000,000 together with the amount of financial protection required. . . .

This means that the operator of a reactor must obtain as much private insurance as he can (the "financial protection required"). The Atomic Energy Commission will then provide $500 million of protection on top of that. (Technically, the AEC "holds harmless" the reator operator for "public liability" up to this amount.) But by law, the reactor operator and the Federal Government *are not liable* for any damages in excess of that $500 million plus private insurance. In other words, if . . . $7 billion in property damage in a single accident . . . [occurred —the maximum as conceived by the AEC], only one-fourteenth of the damage would be covered. This "limitation of liability" clause assures private utilities that no matter how bad an accident is, they will not suffer any financial loss.

The law does provide, however, that utilities owning reactors must buy as much insurance privately as they can. . . . [Two] combines of insurance companies . . . together agreed to provide up to $60 million insurance for each commercial reactor.

It is clear that this is merely a token of private insurance when measured against the government-provided $500 million. Even ten years later, despite constant urging from the Joint Committee [on Atomic Energy], the insurance companies have been only willing to increase their participation to $74 million.

—Novick, *The Careless Atom*, pp. 71–72.

The problem of private participation in the atomic energy program has not improved since 1957, it has grown only worse. The Price-Anderson Act was originally to have run for only ten years. So important is this law for continued private participation in the reactor program that on May 26, 1965, . . . bills [were introduced] in Congress which would extend the law for an additional ten years to 1977, even though it was then still a full two years from expiring. The Joint Committee [on Atomic Energy] held extensive hearings on these bills . . . and discovered that . . . [insurance] companies did not want to take any larger slice of the reactor liability, and utilities would not buy reactors unless [insurance] protection were provided.

. . . Mel Frankel, a nuclear engineer appearing on behalf of the Los Angeles Department of Water and Power . . . testified:

Without the protection, which is presently provided by the Price-Anderson Act, it is doubtful that any utility would consider it prudent to build nuclear plants.

Mr. Frankel also testified that the Department . . . had inserted a clause in its contract to build the Malibu reactor that would allow it to terminate the contract in the event that government or private insurance was not available. "We understand that this provision is standard in most contracts," he said.

This testimony is not reassuring about the confidence of electric utilities in the safety of the reactors they are purchasing in such great numbers.

—Novick, *The Careless Atom*, pp. 73–75.

Used properly, atomic energy might be a valuable force in the civilian as well as the military economy. Reactors can be safe and clean; further research might make them so, at a price that would still allow their use in a competitive economy. The passage of [the] Price-Anderson [Act] has removed the incentive to do the needed research, however, and instead we are developing, not safer, but more dangerous reactors, . . . the hazards of which make even the present plans for huge reactors in the hearts of cities seem tame.

—Novick, *The Careless Atom*, p. 184.

In [May,] 1965, Dr. Edward Teller, often called the "father of the H-Bomb," and not otherwise noted for his caution in advocating the military development of atomic energy, wrote . . . [in the *Journal of Petroleum Technology*]: "In principle, nuclear reactors are dangerous. . . . By being careful, and also by good luck, we have so far avoided all serious nuclear accidents. . . . In my mind, nuclear reactors do not belong on the surface of the earth. Nuclear reactors belong underground."

—Novick, *The Careless Atom*, p. 38.

Underground construction may be an important safety device. It is already in use in Sweden.

—Novick, *The Careless Atom*, p. 186.

Some of us look to technology for salvation and specifically to atomic energy as a source of power. The world's total known supply of low-cost uranium would supply the current US energy needs for only one year. For the last 20 years, the production of nuclear fuel elements has consumed more electrical power than any other user, taking more than 1/10th of all the electrical energy generated.

—"Environmental Quality: Its Significance in Our Environment" (editorial), *JAMA*, Vol. 214, No. 9 (November 30, 1970), p. 1717.

. . . [The] atomic power industry . . . is . . . investing billions upon billions of dollars in atomic power plants on the assumption that cheap fuel will be in supply for the indefinite future.

According to a number of experts, however, *around 1980 we will begin to feel a uranium pinch, and ten years afterward shortages will be critical.* . . .

When the AEC [Atomic Energy Commission] reported on civilian nuclear power to the President in 1962, it . . . felt that after 1980 a [fuel shortage] problem would arise unless the technology for operating breeding reactors, which create more fuel than they burn, was perfected. . . .

Even if breeders do go into operation by 1980, it has been asserted that it will be too late for them to prevent the drain on uranium resources now occurring as a result of soaring orders for conventional reactors. . . .

Whether we manage to satisfy short-term uranium needs or not, the future of atomic energy depends on the breeder. Yet the [technological] problems besetting the breeder program are truly prodigious. . . .

—Curtis and Hogan, *Perils of the Peaceful Atom*, pp. 201–204.

In 1967, Edward Teller [concerning the development of safe, reliable, and economical breeder reactors] stated in *Nuclear News* that "Altogether the fast breeder has resisted the head-on attack of our best technological people for 20 years. I doubt it will become a success very soon." . . .

. . . Edward Teller has described the special dangers of the breeder in these terms:

For the fast breeder to work in its steady-state breeding condition you probably need something like half a ton of plutonium. In order that it should work economically in a sufficiently big power-producing unit, it probably needs quite a bit more than one ton of plutonium. I do not like the hazard involved. I suggested that nuclear reactors are a blessing because they are clean. They *are* clean as long as they function as planned, but if they malfunction in a massive manner, which can happen in principle, they can release enough fission products to kill a tremendous number of people.

. . . [If] you put together two tons of plutonium in a breeder, one tenth of 1 per cent of this material could become critical.

. . . Although I believe it is possible to analyze the immediate consequences of an accident, I do not believe it is possible to analyze and foresee the secondary consequences. In an accident involving a plutonium reactor, a couple of tons of plutonium can melt. I don't think anybody can foresee where 1 or 2 or 5 per cent of this plutonium will find itself and how it will get mixed with some other material. A small fraction of the original charge can become a great hazard.

—Curtis and Hogan, *Perils of the Peaceful Atom*, pp. 206, 209.

The concept of tolerances or acceptable levels of contamination of foodstuffs . . . implies acceptance of the threshold hypothesis. That is to say, for all chemicals there is some level of dosage or concentration, greater than zero, at which there will be no (harmful) effects on exposed individuals. The same concept of the tolerance dose was formerly used in the development of radiation protection standards. In recent years, the accumulation of evidence has cast doubt on the assumption that there is a positive dose that will be safe for all exposed individuals. Evidence on the genetic effects of radiation indicates that extremely small doses delivered to the gonads prior to reproduction will be accompanied by an increase in genetic mutations, most of which are deleterious. The threshold hypothesis has therefore been discarded and an alternative hypothesis accepted that any dose is accompanied by an increased risk of deleterious biological effects, the magnitude of the risk increasing with the dose. The establishment of standards for radiation protection involves balancing the risks inherent in a particular level of exposure against the benefits to be derived.

—J. C. Headley and J. N. Lewis, *The Pesticide Problem: An Economic Approach to Public Policy* (Washington, D.C.: Resources for the Future, 1967), p. 96.

The power problem we face today is not serious enough to warrant precipitous actions that may endanger our future survival. Before the [nuclear power plant] industry builds any more plants, let's set our standards for emissions of radioactive materials at zero. If we do that, we won't have to worry about sources of exposure and changing standards. Let's also require that the cooling water used by the plants be returned in exactly the same condition as when it was taken in. Then we won't have to worry about the amount of damage we will be doing to our waters. The industry doesn't say that this is impossible. It argues that it would be prohibitively expensive, but really that's not up to them. We use the power; we live in the world they pollute. Let them tell us how much it is going to cost and let us make the decision [of] how much survival is worth.

—Ottinger, *What Every Woman Should Know*, p. 36.

FARMINGTON, Conn.—A "little black box" . . . is undergoing a renaissance that could have broad economic and ecological significance.

. . . It's the long-heralded, but still unperfected, "fuel cell," a silent, essentially pollution-free device with no moving parts that produces electricity through a chemical reaction of hydrogen and oxygen. The hydrogen can come from many common fuels—such as natural gas —and the oxygen from the air.

The first field test of a new lower-cost version of the device is under way in a plush display home in this Hartford suburb, and 59 other units will be tested over the next year and a half in . . . diverse locations [around the country]. . . . By the end of next year, its backers, the Pratt & Whitney division of United Aircraft Corp. and 32 gas and electric utilities, will decide whether they will proceed to commercial fuel-cell service by 1975.

If the venture succeeds, its advocates say, it could prove of major benefit in closing the nation's growing energy gap and in tackling some of the most pressing environmental problems. . . .

—Roger W. Benedict, " 'Little Black Box': Fuel Cell, Long Seen as Electricity Source, Moves Ahead in Tests," *The Wall Street Journal* (May 19, 1971), p. 1.

On May 26 [1971], the Scientists' Institute for Public Information (SIPI) filed a complaint in federal court charging the U.S. Atomic Energy Commission with violation of the National Environmental Protection Act. . . . [SIPI has] asked the U.S. District Court of the District of Columbia to require the Atomic Energy Commission to consider alternatives to its program for the development and proliferation of a new type of nuclear power plant, a program which is to cost at least two billion dollars in federal funds. . . .

The program in question is the development and proliferation of the Liquid-Metal-Cooled Fast Breeder (LMFBR), which is a kind of nuclear power plant in which plutonium serves as a fuel. This type of power plant will have a number of serious disadvantages, primarily because of the use of plutonium. . . .

Plutonium is one of the most toxic materials known, and even without a severe accident, the existence of a large number of LMFBRS could result in plutonium contamination of the environment. . . .

. . . [The LMFBR] converts the uranium into plutonium, which is burned as more plutonium is made [by the reactor]. . . .

In the LMFBR . . . , the . . . expensive separation of . . . uranium isotopes is avoided and, presumably, the LMFBR would be able to produce correspondingly cheaper electricity. As a side benefit, reserves of uranium would be conserved.

138

These economic benefits are highly speculative, since the design for a working LMFBR has not been chosen. The first commercial attempt to build such a plant, the Enrico Fermi Nuclear Power Plant near Detroit, Michigan, has been a financial and technical failure. . . .

Assuming that a commercially attractive LMFBR is designed, it will depend on an expanding power industry. . . .

It is by no means necessary or certain that electric power production will continue to grow at present rates . . . [although a] massive federal investment in new power production facilities is a partial assurance that they will be used. . . .

Even assuming the continued growth of electric power production, . . . there are a variety of energy sources which do not suffer from the considerable drawbacks of the LMFBR.

. . . Perhaps the most significant for the long term is the development of fusion reactors, which would not produce the quantities of dangerous wastes associated with today's reactors and the LMFBR. Research and development of fusion reactors have been reduced as a result of the crash program to develop LMFBRS.

The AEC is promoting the LMFBR to an extent unmatched by any other program, public or private, for developing new or improved means for generating electricity. . . .

The National Environmental Protection Act requires the Atomic Energy Commission to consider these alternatives [to the LMFBRS] before proceeding with its program for the commercial development of LMFBRs and to publish its considerations along with its judgment of the environmental impact of the proposed program and alternatives, in a statement to be circulated for public comment and review and to accompany its request for funds from Congress.

SIPI believes it is of the greatest importance that the environmental impact of the LMFBR development program and the alternatives to that program be given full consideration, and has therefore taken legal action to compel the Atomic Energy Commission to do so. [*Environment*] EDITOR's NOTE: After this statement was issued to the press, President Richard M. Nixon announced that the LMFBR development program proposed by the AEC has been adopted as the first priority in his administration's energy policy.

—"Another SST?" *Environment* (July/August 1971), pp. 18–19.

. . . [Knowledgeable] critics have a point in urging a reassessment of the present nuclear program. Though it may eventually fulfill its high promise, there is still time to reevaluate the peaceful atom and make sure that every safeguard has been taken to prevent a tragic misstep.

—"The Peaceful Atom: Friend or Foe," *Time* (January 19, 1970), p. 43.

"The arms race has generally gotten worse in the last 25 years," said . . . George Rathjens, an M.I.T. political scientist. Rathjens, a former Defense Department official and arms control expert, bemoaned what he perceived as the Nixon Administration's renewed interest in nuclear weapons and its revival of the practice of "trying to make policies out of weapons" in a manner similar to U.S. actions at the height of the Cold War in the 1950's. Rathjens spoke of the greater dangers posed by more sophisticated weapons systems; he noted that a single Polaris missile fired accidentally would now destroy a city. In the near future, an accidentally fired Poseidon missile could destroy a dozen cities. Rathjens sounded an alarm about the continued drift on policies governing the use of the many tactical nuclear weapons in Europe, a confusion which could, under the right circumstances, quickly escalate into a general nuclear war. Rathjens argued that people have failed to understand the destructiveness of nuclear weapons. While a government official in the early 1960's, Rathjens said, he looked up a Soviet city the size of Hiroshima and found that a weapon fully 200 times as powerful as the Hiroshima bomb had been targeted for the Soviet city by the Defense Department.

—Bryce Nelson, "Hiroshima after 25 Years: 'We Are All Survivors'," *Science*, Vol. 171, No. 3971 (February 12, 1971), p. 556.

WASHINGTON, Oct. 11—Substantial numbers of Americans may be doomed to live lives of mediocrity because of minor and undetectable damage they sustained before they were born, a pioneer in radiation protection research suggested today.

The researcher, Dr. Karl Z. Morgan, director of the Health Physics Division of Oak Ridge National Laboratory, cited this as one of the penalties the nation might incur because of laxity in its use of medical X-rays.

Dr. Morgan testified before a House subcommittee considering radiation problems.

The scientist said exposure of Americans to X-rays could be cut to 10 per cent of its present level without lowering the quality or amount of diagnostic information. In fact, he said, the quality and quantity can be improved while the total dose is being drastically reduced.

"These hearings are for the purpose of reducing population exposure to all forms of man-made sources of ionizing radiation," said Dr. Morgan. "Since over 90 per cent of all exposure in the United States to man-made sources of ionizing radiation results from medical exposure and most of this is from medical diagnosis, it follows that unnecessary or wasteful diagnostic exposure should be our first concern at these hearings."

Many animal studies have proved that exposure of the fetus in the womb to X-rays can produce birth defects, including crippling, impaired vision and mental retardation. Extreme doses of X-rays can be fatal.

Dr. Morgan said that there was also evidence that the death rate from leukemia and other forms of cancer was 40 per cent higher in children who had been exposed to X-rays before they were born than it was in children not exposed.

He continued:

"There is some evidence that for every detectable form of damage there may be 10,000 other forms of somatic, and probably genetic, damage which go undetected throughout the life of the individual but nevertheless represent a serious burden as he attempts to compete for an equal place in our modern society and perhaps never attains the highest stages of efficiency and excellence because of some form of damage that had its origin during fetal development." . . .

Many radiation specialists agree that it is unwise to X-ray a pregnant woman unless some grave danger to her or to the baby requires it.

Nevertheless, Dr. Morgan said, it is estimated that at least 22 per cent of all pregnant women have one or more X-ray examinations and, in 10 per cent, the X-rays are aimed at the lower abdomen—the area in which the fetus is most likely to be hit.

—Harold M. Schmeck Jr., "Scientist Links Mediocrity to Fetuses Damaged in Lax X-Ray Examinations," *The New York Times* (October 12, 1967), p. 35.

. . . [Addressing a House subcommittee on Oct. 11, Dr. Karl Z. Morgan] estimated that continued use of X-rays at the present rate in a population of the nation's current size could lead to as many as 27,000 deaths a year from genetic defects; 1,100 from leukemia and a non-specific life-shortening effect to 1,000 persons.

No such calculations could ever be proved because the deaths would be indistinguishable from others . . . that presumably were not caused by radiation effects. The calculations are based on animal experiments and on the results of exposures of both men and animals to much higher doses than are ever given during diagnostic X-ray use.

—Harold M. Schmeck Jr., "Caution on X-Ray-'Don't Overdo It'," *The New York Times* (October 15, 1967), The Week in Review section, p. 6.

Commenting on the prevention of cancer [*The Lancet*, 1967], we suggested that one of the many pressing reasons for increasing efforts in this direction is that cancer is now a main cause of death in childhood. . . .

. . . A [large] prospective investigation by MacMahon in the United States [*Journal of the National Cancer Institute*, Vol. 28 (1962), p. 1173] demonstrated that the excess risk of obstetric radiography was of the order of 1.3 to 1.5 percent. Thus, there now seems little doubt that X-rays may cause an excess risk in the development of cancer in the offspring of mothers exposed during pregnancy.

Dr. Alice Stewart and Mr. G. W. Kneale have extended the earlier work to see whether changes in the practice of obstetric radiography have altered the development of cancer in children [*The Lancet*, Vol. I (January 28, 1968), p. 104]. . . . Stewart and Kneale suggest that 5.5 % of all the cases of cancer in childhood were due to obstetric radiography . . . [and] show that at the beginning of the study period [covering 1943 to 1965] children who were exposed to X-rays were over twice as likely to die from cancer as were their non-exposed contemporaries, while at the end of the period of study this risk was only 1.4 times as great.

—"X-Rays and Childhood Cancer" (editorial), *The Lancet*, 1968, Vol. I (March 16, 1968), pp. 577–78.

Epidemiological data from the Oxford Survey of Childhood Cancers has been analysed in respect of in-utero exposure to X-rays during obstetric investigations. The risk of cancer was greatest when exposure was during the first trimester. The excess cancer risk from obstetric X-ray examination was directly related to the fetal dose. It is suggested that this dose-response relationship fits in with a previously published hypothesis that cancers caused in this way are due to the propagation of one cell whose controlling gene had experienced a small but irreversible change at the moment of exposure to X-rays.

—Alice Stewart and G. W. Kneale, "Radiation Dose Effects in Relation to Obstetric X-Rays and Childhood Cancers," *The Lancet,* 1970, Vol. II (June 6, 1970), p. 1185.

A four-year study of 216 families with children who have Down's syndrome (mongoloid idiocy) shows that the mothers had a significant excess exposure to both fluoroscopic and therapeutic irradiation prior to the birth of the child.

More surprising, the study indicates an increase in radar exposure in a significant number of fathers of the mongoloid children.

A report of the study was read to the annual meeting of the American Public Health Association by Arnold T. Sigler, MD, instructor, Department of Pediatrics, Johns Hopkins School of Medicine. Co-authors were Abraham M. Lilienfeld MD, Bernice H. Cohen, PhD, and Jeannette E. Westlake, RN.

Families included in the study were matched with control families of normal children by sex of the child and date and place of birth.

Mothers of the mongoloid children had approximately seven times as much exposure to irradiation from one or more diagnostic, fluoroscopic, and therapeutic sources as did the mothers of controls. In addition, significantly fewer mothers of children with Down's syndrome had not received any radiation prior to birth of the children.

These findings, Dr. Sigler said, are "consistent with the views concerning cumulative radiation damage to genetic material."

"These results strongly suggest that maternal ionizing radiation exposure may be one etiological factor responsible for some cases of mongolism," Dr. Sigler said. He emphasized, however, that this may be only one of several important factors in the pathogenesis of the condition.

He described the suggested relationship between Down's

syndrome and paternal radar exposure as "puzzling."

"The increased radar exposure of fathers of mongols as compared with controls raises the question as to whether ionizing radiation, in addition to the known heating effect, may be involved in radar operations," he said.

"Since, however, no greater exposure to medical radiation was observed among fathers of mongols as compared to fathers of controls, radar, under special circumstances, must involve some unique and potent effect that overcomes the male advantage of continuous spermatogenesis," Dr. Sigler concluded.

> —"Radiation and Radar Exposure Implicated in Down's Syndrome," *JAMA*, Vol. 194 (November 1, 1965), p. 34.

DENVER, Oct. 27—A study of birth and death records in the Grand Junction, Colo., area where radioactive sands from uranium processing mills were used in construction projects, shows increased genetic problems, higher cancer rates and lower birth rates than those of the rest of the state.

These findings were disclosed in remarks prepared for presentation tomorrow to the Raw Materials Subcommittee of the Congressional Joint Committee on Atomic Energy in Washington. Dr. C. Henry Kempe and Dr. Robert M. Ross Jr. said, "These differences could be attributable to radiation." . . .

Dr. Kempe is chairman of the department of pediatrics at the University of Colorado School of Medicine here, and Dr. Ross is a practicing pediatrician in Grand Junction and surrounding Mesa County.

The two men were part of a six-man medical advisory committee appointed by the Colorado Department of Health, which recommended removal of the radioactive sand, called mill tailings, from homes, businesses, offices, schools, churches and public buildings in Grand Junction. Abnormally high radiation readings have been found at almost 6,500 locations in 11 Colorado cities and towns. The largest number of readings, 4,984, were found in the Grand Junction area in western Colorado. . . .

Because of the low levels involved, the effects of such radiation are seldom immediate, sometimes taking as long as 20 or 30 years to develop. . . .

In their prepared testimony, the two physicians said the decision by the medical committee to recommend removal of all tailings was based in part on the study of birth and death records.

The study, they said, showed that the rate of deaths caused by congenital irregularities from 1965 to 1968 was 8.2 cases per 1,000 births in Mesa County, compared with 5.2 cases per 1,000 births in the state. In the last 10 years, the frequency of such deaths has increased slightly in Mesa County, while declining in the state as a whole, they reported.

Cleft lips and cleft palates, both genetic problems, were almost twice as common in Mesa County during the same period: 2.2 cases per 1,000 births, compared with 1.2 cases statewide, the doctors said.

They also reported that birth rates were "significantly lower" in Mesa County during the same period: 14.5 per 1,000 in Mesa County and 17.9 per 1,000 statewide.

The pediatricians also found that the over-all rate of deaths caused by cancer was "significantly higher" from 1965 to 1969: Mesa County had 153 cases per 100,000 population, versus 123 cases per 100,000 statewide. . . .

—Anthony Ripley, "Radioactive Sands Linked to Higher Death Rates," *The New York Times*, Oct. 28, 1971, p. 27

GRAND JUNCTION, Colo., Sept. 30—The spotlights have come down again on this city on the western slope of the Rocky Mountains over the widespread use of radioactive sands in building projects.

The state government is aroused and calling for Federal action. The Joint Congressional Committee on Atomic Energy is planning hearings on possible health hazards. A state-Federal steering committee has recommended removal of the radioactive material from habitable buildings.

But, out of sight, away from the center stage where the politicians and bureaucrats play out their public roles, stands a worried small-town doctor who has started a quiet campaign to see if the dangers of radioactivity to human health can actually be measured in Grand Junction.

Dr. Robert M. Ross Jr. practices children's medicine. . . . He is

145

past president of the Mesa County Medical Association, a respected man.

Like most people in Grand Junction, he has known for some time that radioactive sands—called "tailings," which were dumped in piles back of the Climax Uranium Company ore-processing mill—have been spread all over town. . . .

. . . [The] radioactivity comes right up through the concrete in the form of a gas called radon and that radon is blamed by medical experts for the high rates of lung cancer among uranium miners.

Many in town dismissed the problem as distortion by the press —and some still do, despite the latest flurry of attention.

But Dr. Ross was not among them.

Watching the patients come into his office, he was troubled by what he calls a vague sense that something was not right. He said he was seeing too many birth defects, too much cancer in children. . . .

"When questions about the tailings really came up about two years ago," he said, "I began to wonder if it really was a problem."

He began to take extra notice of cases of blood, muscle and nerve cancer and of birth defects; mongolism and premature fusion of the skull bones of infants.

"There is no proof," he added. "Even with the number of children with malignancies and genetic anomalies, the figures were not really beyond what one should expect."

But he couldn't shake the worry from his mind.

He spoke of his concern to Dr. C. Henry Kempe, chairman of the pediatrics department at the University of Colorado Medical Center in Denver.

Dr. Kempe and his associates went to the Colorado Department of Health with the problem and it was thrown onto the agenda of a meeting arranged with Gov. John A. Love last March. At the meeting were three representatives of the State Health Department and six from the Atomic Energy Commission.

They reviewed other atomic matters in the state and when the indoor radon problem came up, the State Health Department suggested that the A.E.C. finance a chromosomal study of infants in Grand Junction.

One of those at the meeting remembered that the A.E.C. response was negative, that the representatives argued that there was no evidence to begin with, that the radon levels were too low and that there were too few births in Grand Junction for the study to have any statistical significance.

Ever former A.E.C. Chairman Glenn T. Seaborg later wrote Governor Love turning the grant request down.

But the State Health Department persisted and persuaded the Governor to spend $18,000 from his special research and studies fund to finance the project.

Work began in July and involves chromosomal studies of infants born during 1971. About 700 babies a year are born in Grand Junction. Comparisons are being made between infants conceived and carried until birth in homes built on tailings and those from homes free from the radioactive sands.

Dr. Herbert Lubs, a geneticist with the university medical center, is doing the study and said no results would be known until next year.

But another source close to the study said that chromosomal abnormalities not usually found in infants were being discovered.

"We're concerned not so much with adults as with possible genetic damage to their grandchildren," Dr. Kempe said. . . . "It's not this generation of parents but their children's children." . . .

—Anthony Ripley, "Infants and Radioactive Sands: Small-Town Doctor Wins Fight," The New York Times, October 3, 1971, p. 75.

Harmful effects of ionizing radiation on the developing fetus were noted during the early days of radiation therapy. In 1929 Goldstein and Murphy reported that large doses of radiation to the pelvic region of pregnant women sometimes resulted in microcephaly in the offspring [L. Goldstein and D. C. Murphy, in *American Journal of Roentgenology*, Vol. 22 (October 1929), pp. 322–31]. More recently, it has been suggested that diagnostic irradiation during the prenatal period may result in an increased incidence of leukemia in the exposed children [A. Stewart, J. Webb, and D. Hewitt, in *British Medical Journal*, Vol. 1 (June 28, 1958), pp. 1495–1508]. With these findings in mind, special attention has been directed to a group of children who were exposed in utero to ionizing radiation from the atomic bomb in Hiroshima and Nagasaki. These children, along with suitable control groups, have been observed as part of a long-term study of the delayed

147

effects of the atomic bomb. Early studies revealed an increased incidence of microcephaly and mental retardation.

. . . Burrow et al report another and more subtle aspect of the dangers of prenatal irradiation in the atomic bomb group [G. Burrow et al, in *JAMA*, vol. 192, No. 5 (May 3, 1965), pp. 357–64]. Children exposed in utero lagged behind nonexposed peers during adolescence in several aspects of growth and development. With few exceptions the exposed children could be considered individually within "normal limits" in terms of growth and development. The differences became apparent only when a suitable control group was used for comparison. These findings suggest that, in addition to easily recognized abnormalities, irradiation in utero may result in more subtle defects such as a failure to achieve optimal growth and development. There is no reason to think these effects are limited solely to nuclear irradiation. Certainly, microcephaly has occurred as an aftermath of both nuclear and X-irradiation. The lag in growth and development was most pronounced in children whose mothers had received a radiation dose of 50 rad or more. However, there is no convincing evidence that a threshold exists for radiation effects, and it is likely that smaller amounts of radiation might cause even more subtle changes.

The thalidomide tragedy has focused attention on a variety of agents which are tolerated by the mother but harmful to the fetus. Prenatal irradiation can be such an agent. The results of the present study suggest that radiation effects may occur which are detrimental to the fetus but are not readily apparent. These effects which are difficult to detect constitute another compelling reason to avoid unnecessary irradiation of the fetus during pregnancy.

—"Irradiation in Utero" (editorial), *JAMA*, Vol. 192, No. 5, (May 3, 1965), p. 410.

Benign thyroid nodules were removed from three teenage Rongelap girls ten years after . . . [accidental exposure to fallout radiation following the detonation of a high-yield U.S. nuclear device at Bikini, on March 1, 1954.] (The thyroid dose received was estimated at about 1,000 rads, largely from radioiodines absorbed.) No thyroid nodules were detected in 75 unexposed children. Other possible residual radiation effects noted in the 86 exposed Rongelapese were as follows: slight retardation of statural growth and bone maturation in boys exposed at less than 5 years of age; greater incidence of miscarriages in exposed women during the first four years; incomplete recovery of some of the peripheral blood elements; and increased nevus-like lesions in areas of previous beta radiation burns of the skin. General health and mortality has been about the same as in the comparison population. No definite radiation effects on birth rate, aging, leukemia, malignancy, or geno-type have been noted.

—Robert A. Conard and Arobati Hicking, (abstract of) "Medical Findings in Mar-shallese People Exposed to Fallout Radiation," *JAMA*, Vol. 192, No. 6 (May 10, 1965), p. 457.

Cytogenetic studies of blood lymphocytes of Marshall Islanders, 10 years after their [accidental] exposure to radiation from fallout in 1954, show chromosome-type aberrations in 23 of 43 exposed persons. Half the aberrations are of the exchange type. An unexpectedly large number of acentric fragments, but no exchange-type aberrations, appear in a few unexposed people on the same island [Rongelap Island].

—Hermann Lisco and Robert A. Conard, (abstract of) "Chromosome Studies on Marshall Islanders Exposed to Fallout Radiation," *Science*, Vol. 157, No. 3787 (July 28, 1967), p. 445.

Roentgen [X-ray] therapy has been used for many years in patients with adolescent acne vulgaris. Without proper shielding of the neck the thyroid gland may receive undetermined amounts of irradiation. The potential carcinogenic effect on the thyroid has largely been ignored by the therapist in this group of patients, although the association of thyroid cancer and irradiation to the thymus in infancy is well recognized. . . .

Five adult patients with thyroid cancer, in whom it was possible to obtain a history of radiation therapy for acne vulgaris in adolescence, have been seen. . . .

. . . [They] were treated for acne vulgaris during middle to late adolescence with ionizing radiation not directed at the thyroid, and thyroid cancer developed in each after several years' time. Because a causal relationship between incidental radiation to the thyroid and carcinogenesis cannot be disproved, radiation therapy for acne and other benign diseases of the head and neck should be abandoned in the adolescent patient.

—Edwin C. Albright and Robert W. Allday, "Thyroid Carcinoma After Radiation Therapy for Adolescent Acne Vulgaris," *JAMA*, Vol. 199, No. 4 (January 23, 1967), pp. 280–81.

J. A. Haybittle of the Radiotherapeutic Center at Addenbrooke's Hospital in Cambridge, England, has reported in *Nature* (17 May 1958) that some luminous-dial wrist watches contain sufficient radium to subject their owners to nearly two-thirds the maximum permissible level for [radiation] exposure of hands and forearms. According to Haybittle, one watch having an estimated radium content of 2.2 μc [microcuries] recorded on a film placed in contact with the back of the watch a dose rate of 8 mr/hr [milliroentgens per hour].

During the past year we have been investigating the degree of radioactivity of luminous-dial wrist watches. . . . Watches were found to vary more than tenfold in their [radiation] activity. . . .

With an activity of 8 mr/hr at a distance of 8 in. a wrist watch worn 24 hours a day can deliver 1.1 r [roentgens] a year; this is the dosage that might be delivered to the gonads by the most active watches when the watch is worn on the wrist in a position facing the gonads. The least active watches would deliver approximately one-tenth of this activity. . . . The potentially harmful magnitude of the radiation from the most active watches, corresponding to 5 rem in about 5 years, may be judged in the light of the recommendation by the International Committee on Radiation Protection that no one should receive a dose in excess of 5 rem by age 30.

When one further considers that this radiation is several times greater than natural background radiation and exceeds by more than 100 times that presently received from radioactive fallout, the potential hazard to the wearer of a luminous-dial wrist watch raises the question as to whether the small benefit that may be received from such a watch is worth the hazard.

—Grafton D. Chase and Arthur Osol (School of Chemistry, Philadelphia College of Pharmacy and Science) (letter), *Science*, Vol. 128, No. 3327 (October 3, 1958), p. 788.

The first comparison [of radiodiagnostic examinations] is with the wearing of a typical radium-dial wrist watch. . . . The calculated dose to the gonads *per annum* [from such a watch can be conservatively estimated at] 20 mr *per annum.* . . .

. . . [The] number of radiographic examinations . . . that an individual may accept before the gonad dose (genetic hazard) equals that received from the average radium-dial wrist watch worn for ten years . . . [is such that], if the testicles are protected from direct exposure in examinations. . . , several such examinations may be given before the hazard exceeds that of wearing the watch; more than 1,000 chest or skull examinations may be given.

—Edward W. Webster, "Hazards of Diagnostic Radiology: A Physicist's Point of View," *Radiology,* Vol. 72, No. 4 (April 1959), p. 498.

During the year 1959 a Swiss watch manufacturer marketed wrist-watches with luminous dials painted with a compound marked under the trade name of Lumostabil. After wearing these watches for several weeks, a number of persons were treated for burns on their wrists corresponding to the circle of luminous figures. Lumostabil, which was sold without any warning of its radioactivity, merely happened to contain a large amount of strontium 90! One woman wore such a watch for eight weeks. It is believed to have been illuminated with about 20 microcuries of strontium 90. It is estimated that this woman received a cumulative dose of 10.15 thousand rad. The radiation dose from contact with the front of the watch might have been about 10 rad per hour! In December 1959 several such watches, apparently illuminated with the same compound, were recalled by their vendors in the United States.

In November 1962 the New York City Board of Health banned the sale of radium-dial pocket watches. Studies by the Health Department's Office of Radiation Control had revealed that the radium-dial pocket watches emitted 75 radiation units a year. This is 150 times more than the permissible or safe amount of 0.5 units a year.

—E. W. Robinson, *The Use of Radium in Consumer Products* (Washington, D.C.: Government Printing Office, 1968).

Gold jewelry may be contaminated sufficiently with radiation to represent a hazard to the wearer. The finding of gold rings containing decay products of radon has prompted this report. . . .

Radon 222, an inert gas, is a daughter element of radium 226. The gas is compressed into a tiny gold tube or seed for use in implantation of tumors. . . . [The] decay products of radon . . . deposit on gold and . . . may remain active enough to cause superficial skin reactions for many years. The gold of the wedding rings [of the two patients examined] . . . contained decayed radon seeds or gold tubing containing unused and decayed radon from a radon plant. Further, the gold had not been refined; during this process the radon deposit would have been separated.

. . . [Not] all gold handlers are . . . equipped to detect radiation, and it is reasonable to assume that contaminated gold has escaped into the jewelry market. This assumption warrants investigation into observations made by jewelers that some people can wear one type of gold, but another "type" irritates the skin. . . .

When unexplained skin reaction results from contact with gold jewelry, radiation reaction should be suspected, and the gold should be tested for radioactivity. Gold to be processed for jewelry and dental use should be monitored for radiation contamination with gold seeds of decayed radon.

—Norman Simon and John Harley, "Skin Reactions From Gold Jewelry Contaminated With Radon Deposit," *JAMA*, Vol. 200, No. 3 (April 17, 1967), pp. 254–55.

Microwave radiation is defined as that part of the electromagnetic energy spectrum lying between 300 and 300,000 megacycles/sec, corresponding to wavelengths between 1 meter and 1 mm. Radar transmitters, long-distance telephone and television communications relay systems, medical diathermic equipment, and certain devices for rapid cooking utilize this type of radiant energy.

—David S. Rosenthal and Steven C. Beering, "Hypogonadism After Microwave Radiation," *JAMA*, Vol 205, No. 4 (July 22, 1968), p. 245.

This paper reports, to our knowledge, the first case in which microwaves appear to have been a factor in the induction of male infertility, without demonstrable improvement 11 months after the first exposure. . . .

A 31-year-old white man, the father of a 4-year-old child, was . . . a repairman at a weather radar installation where he had been employed for four years. He frequently performed maintainance on the radar antenna while the equipment was in operation. . . .

Our patient was exposed repeatedly to microwave power densities more than 3,000 times the currently accepted safe level established by the US Air Force (USAF standards: maximum permissible power density for continous exposure is 10 mw [milliwatts]/sq cm, for brief exposure 100 mw/sq cm). Such exposure raises the question of biologic damage.

> —Rosenthal and Beering, "Hypogonadism After Microwave Radiation," *JAMA* (July 22, 1968), pp. 246–47.

. . . That microwave ovens are manufactured to stringent safety standards does not make them harmless. Although these appliances have been used since 1950 without reported injuries, recently it has been discovered that the initial signs of microwave cataract are asymptomatic and may not appear until years after the exposure has occurred. Further, if the patient delays obtaining an eye examination until he has failing vision, the etiological signs may be masked at that time by cataractous changes in the lens substance. Before accepting the idea that no injuries are attributable from ovens, we should be given evidence that specific types of microwave injury were sought and found to be absent.

The best method to express permissible microwave exposure is in terms of 10 milliwatts/sq cm, the standard used for occupational environments. . . . [More] than 400 of the microwave workers whom I examined had known exposures exceeding 10 milliwatts/sq cm and 41 of the microwave cataract cases I have seen came from this pool.

> —Milton M. Zaret, M.D. (letter), *JAMA*, Vol. 217, No. 4 (July 26, 1971), pp. 481–82.

7

Noise Pollution

❋

"The highest degree of earthly happiness," said Dr. Johnson, "is quiet." What an un-American idea! But then, Dr. Johnson was an Englishman, and anyway lived in the eighteenth century. . . . It may be recalled that during that period Schopenhauer wrote an essay "On Noise," in which he bitterly complained of the . . . [mind-shattering] cracking of coachmen's whips and other objectionable contemporary eruptions of noise. Schopenhauer added that "the amount of noise which anyone can bear undisturbed stands in inverse proportion to his mental capacity, and may therefore be regarded as a pretty fair measure of it." What would Schopenhauer have thought of the noises perpetrated by the modern . . . driver [of motor vehicles], the honking of horns, the [ear-splitting] backfiring [of engines], [the] screeching, groaning, [and] swishing of automobiles, trucks, and buses, the . . . [intolerable] infernal [unthrottled] roaring and staccato of motorcycles, the whining [and droning] of jet aircraft, and the sonic boom [of military planes]? . . .

This "stench in the ear," as Ambrose Bierce called it, these destructive unwanted sounds, are appropriately coming to be called [what they are,] noise pollution.

—Adapted by Montagu, from his book *The American Way of Life*, pp. 122–23.

[Quiet and privacy are reservations] . . . of civilized life which Americans do not . . . [rate very highly]. Hence, high walls, green hedges, or fences do not separate them from their neighbors. . . . [Picture windows are not so much, it would seem, designed for one to look out as for others to look in.] Mowing the lawn [with a machine equipped with the loudest of internal combustion engines] at all sorts of hours disturbing to one's neighbors—were those neighbors disturbable, is considered, if it is considered at all, [the] . . . right of every homeowner, [for] . . . that last infirmity of the suburban mind, the manicured lawn, the pride that only too often goes before the fall, is the occasion of all those pesticides and weed poisons, powders and potions which are thought-lessly injected into the air for one's neighbors to take into their lungs, whether they desire to do so or not. The children [whoop] . . . all over the place, shouting at the tops of their voices, they grow up to be so fond of noise that they come to identify [loudness] . . . with gaiety. If foreigners find Americans objectionably noisy, it is because they fail to understand that Americans do not consider that they are really having a good time unless there is a certain amount of noise associated with it. To Americans, noise is neither irksome nor disagreeable, as it is in other countries, but a reassurance that while there is noise, there is life.

—Adapted by Montagu, from his book *The American Way of Life*, p. 121.

Loud-voiced Americans are not oppressed by loud noises. It is [not that one] seldom . . . hears a quiet-voiced American[, but that there are far too many loud-voiced ones—a fact that foreigners are always noticing and commenting upon.] Conversations in public vehicles are [only too often] . . . conducted as if everyone else were an audience. . . . A loud voice . . . betrays a shallow mind. America has no monopoly on shallow minds, but it does seem to have a very large proportion of loudmouths. . . . The loudmouths are by no means restricted to the uneducated and the underprivileged. . . . [, for] it seems to be a point among many who should know better to make their presence felt by their raucous voices and [crass] . . . disregard for the privacy of others, as if to make it clear how much they think of themselves and how little [of] . . . others. That [loud] talk can be noise and an irritating invasion of privacy never seems to occur to them—these contributors to the [noxiousness of the air]. . . .

—Adapted by Montagu, from his book *The American Way of Life*, pp. 123–24.

The private poisoners of the atmosphere and disturbers of the peace make possible the public enemies of quietude. Among the chief [of these] offenders are the public-address systems which assault one's [ears] . . . with their abominations, without as much as a by-your-leave. Up and down the streets mobile public-address units [,] usually announcing the dubious virtues of a candidate for political office, are permitted to break in on one wherever one may be, one's home being no more sacrosanct than the open street. And not only from the streets but also from airborne vehicles the curse of Babel may descend on one [,] so that there is no escape. And when it is not noise to which one is being subjected, these vehicles will either write their crapulous eructations in the skies or drag the lettered advertising behind them like some pennant announcing the edge of doom.

—Adapted by Montagu, from his book *The American Way of Life*, p. 124.

State and city authorities are no less guilty [than the private contributors to the elevation of] . . . the decibel count of noise. Such public agencies are among the most barbarous and inconsiderate of offenders. Their licensed noises [constitute] . . . sanctioned iniquities. Are not the piercing shrieks of police sirens an offense unto the spirit of man? What is their purpose? I have always assumed that it was in most cases an act of consideration on the part of the police designed to apprise criminals of their impending arrival so that the criminals might have plenty of time to make a leisurely getaway. [Most other] . . . countries somehow contrive to manage these matters much more quietly and effectively. If a police car requires a right of way, surely there are superior means to announcing the official need for the right of way? Fire trucks, rescue squad cars, and ambulances—all are offenders. Surely a signaling system could be easily devised, with every car equipped with the necessary device which would enable official cars to announce their needs?

—Adapted by Montagu, from his book *The American Way of Life*, p. 125.

The introduction of the trolley cars into the larger cities is not only an encroachment upon private rights of the inhabitants, but the whole management of such ponderous machines, through the crude and unscientific principle of construction, is not only a waste of force, but its practical application becomes a veritable nuisance. Such a method of conducting travel we have reason to fear will to a very great extent continue to be so, on account of the insufferable noises that must necessarily result from the operating of such cars by the companies for the sole purpose evidently of gain. Such harsh, bewildering sounds, such fiendish, hideous clangor with which the ears of the would-be sleeper must ever ring, can not but act injuriously upon his whole organism. Though legislative enactments thus far have not been put forth in the direction to lead to the abatement of the evil, yet there is no sufficient reason why the State should not take cognizance of any factor that may disturb to such a degree the health and comfort of mankind.

—"Control of Noises," *JAMA* (September 14, 1895); reprinted in JAMA, Vol. 213, No. 11 (Sept. 14, 1970), p. 1771.

Anxiety, constrained and explosive rage, disturbed sleep, irritability, and concentration and energy draining tensions, are direct and preventable results of noise in our community.

—*Toward a Quieter City*, The Mayor's Task Force on Noise Control (New York, 1970), p. 23.

Today's population is about eight times that of 1850 but produces thirty-five times as much. In putting forth this great rise in material goods it also produces, as a by-product, thirty-five times as much noise. And whereas in 1850 only 15 percent of the people were submitted to production's bang-and-clatter, today 70 per cent of the people are so afflicted.

—Robert Rienow and Leona Train Rienow, *Moment in the Sun* (New York-Dial, 1967), p. 149.

Noise in the areas of America where most people live is twice as loud today as it was fifteen years ago. This attack upon our physical and nervous systems may double again in the next ten to fifteen years unless we pay careful and concerted attention to techniques for muffling the machinery of our industrial civilization.

—Henry Still, *In Quest of Quiet* (Harrisburg, Pa.: Stackpole Books, 1970), p. 9.

In layman's parlance the word "noisy" is applied to any sound that makes it difficult to speak or to be heard. By this standard 80 decibels is considered "loud," 100 decibels labeled "deafening," and anything over 120 decibels is "dangerously high."

—Rienow and Rienow, *Moment in the Sun*, p. 141.

In London, a survey of residents showed traffic to be the most serious annoyance of all sound sources.

According to Prof. William Burns of the University of London, the survey showed that the highest noise levels are associated with buses and heavy goods vehicles, with occasional motorcycles and sports cars. The heavy diesel-engined commercial vehicle is the main source of noise, and noise seems to be a built-in feature of these vehicles. In view of the similarity of design on a world-wide basis, this is an important technical problem with very wide consequences.

—Still, *In Quest of Quiet*, p. 63.

Quieter vehicles will be obtained only when a quieter and more efficient power source provides an economic successor to the diesel and gasoline engines.

—Still, *In Quest of Quiet*, p. 70.

Is Boston really noisy? To find out, this reporter — decibel meter in hand — poked around the city one afternoon in search of noisemakers. . . .

A big jetliner registered 103 decibels as it soared over the Prudential tower. It was about 1,200 feet up and the meter was on the street.

. . . [Two] motorcycles, sans mufflers, . . . zoomed down apartment-lined Beacon Street. They jolted the gauge to 107 decibels inside a third-floor residence.

Jackhammers measured 98 decibels at 10 feet and rose to 123 decibels from the workman's vantage point two feet from the yammering chisel.

—Jack Dillon, "Researchers Wrestle Challenge of City Noise," *The Christian Science Monitor* (September 13, 1965), p. 13.

Millions of Americans today live with 100-dB noise levels where homes and apartments are built within 200 feet of a busy downtown street or expressway. . . . Most people remain indoors most of the time and thus are protected from ear-damaging sound from road traffic, which, with a wall to attenuate it, may fall to 70 or 80 dB.

—Still, *In Quest of Quiet*, p. 62.

161

Russian investigators blame sounds of . . . [about the] 50 dB . . . [level] for making falling asleep a lengthy process, of about an hour and a half. Deep sleep which followed lasted only an hour; this was followed, on awakening, by "a sense of fatigue accompanied by palpitations." (Noise hangover?) The fairly quiet level of 35 dB, the Russians found, was the threshold for optimum sleeping conditions.

—Theodore Berland, *The Fight for Quiet,* (Englewood Cliffs, N.J.: Prentice-Hall, 1970), pp. 68–69.

Recent research has shown that sleep, accompanied by dreaming, is essential to mental health. Dr. Jerome Lukas, psychologist at Stanford Research Institute, looked into . . . [the problem of how noise affects sleep] and found that his volunteer dreamers, subjected to noise while sleeping, woke up extremely fatigued. Dr. Lukas concluded that this fatigue was caused by the effort to maintain sleep in spite of the noise. The close relationship between that fatigue and that noise suggested that a sleeping person suffers from noise even when it is not so intense as to awaken him.

—*Toward a Quieter City,* p. 14.

America has some of the finest hotels [and motels] in the world [,] and some of the worst—the newest ones . . . especially. . . . [The] new hotels . . . [usually have such thin uninsulated walls and floors that every voice and every step is immediately transmitted, as well as the crackling of TV, the radio, and telephone. The bathroom noises might just as well be in the middle of one's own room, and as for the flushing toilets, these] . . . disturb one's sleep and give one nightmares, for when a toilet is flushed it sounds like the combined [thundering] . . . of the cataracts of the Nile and the Victoria and Niagara Falls—louder, in fact, for water seems to be rushing straight through the walls . . . [to engulf one's hapless body]. What single mindlessness it must have taken to have planned such comforts for . . . [prospective guests? The truth is no one gave these potential disturbers of the peace a moment's thought, for Americans are not consciously bothered by such disturbances, since noise is the daily accompaniment of their lives].

[But worse than all these noises combined are the high frequency low intensity sounds made by various motors which principally serve

162

the air-conditioning units in these newer hostelries. One may succeed in turning off the air-conditioning in the room, but the noises from the motors cannot be turned off, and, indeed, have a way of becoming amplified the moment the traveler puts his head on the pillow. Ear plugs cannot shut the noise out, nor can locking oneself in the closet or bathroom—the noise is pervasive. And it is enough to drive one mad —and, I daresay, in the course of time it would—but not most Americans; they don't notice it, even though they may feel fatigued after a night with such "humming."]

—Adapted by Montagu, from his book *The American Way of Life*, p. 309.

H. R. Richter of Basel, Switzerland, studied the brain waves (electroencephalograms or EEG) of sleepers and concluded that "noise associated with modern civilization (automobiles, trucks, elevated and underground railways, jets) and even natural sounds (birds, etc.) frequently disturb the rest of sleepers" without their usually being aware of this. This finding agrees with that of Dr. Gerd Jansen in Germany, who found that similarly moderate noises had their definite effects on sleepers' physiology. "All sounds audible at night impair the quality of sleep," in his view.

—Berland, *The Fight for Quiet*, p. 67.

Julius Buchwald, M.D., psychiatrist with the Downstate Division of the New York State Medical Center, said [in reporting on what can happen to people noisily deprived of sleep] that interruption of dreams can lead to psychotic symptoms ranging from mild to severe. Among these are nightmarish memories, paranoidal delusions, hallucinations, and suicidal and homicidal tendencies. . . . Noise, further, can reduce one's sense of humor and ability to handle ordinary, everyday frustrations.

—Berland, *The Fight for Quiet*, p. 69.

One of the major reasons why noise in the home has become a serious and growing problem, although it seems paradoxical in this age of advanced affluence and technology, is that homes (including apartments) are not built as well as they used to be. . . . As stated by the

163

Committee on Environmental Quality [of the Federal Council for Science and Technology, in September 1968]:

"Many of the old-fashioned dwellings of 40 or 50 years ago . . . were comparatively quiet places in which to live. In contrast, the modern dwelling with its light-weight construction, open plan design and multitude of noise makers provides very little protection from noise generated within or intruding from the clamorous outdoors. . . ."

—Still, *In Quest of Quiet*, p. 25.

. . . [The] United States is one of the few major nations in the world which does not have regulations setting minimum requirements for the insulation of buildings against sound.

—Still, *In Quest of Quiet*, p. 27.

Exposure to excessive and sustained noise can cause . . . loss of hearing, sometimes permanently. Researchers estimate that a minimum of six to sixteen million industrial workers sustain degrees of hearing loss from exposure to noise on the job. Nationally, claims for compensation because of hearing loss amount annually to two million dollars.

—*Toward a Quieter City*, p. 14.

Ideally, noise control will be achieved in industry when buildings are designed initially with low sound levels in mind, and *additionally* designed with noise-controlled machinery placed in proper locations.

—Still, *In Quest of Quiet*, p. 152.

. . . [In California] in the 12 months ending last June 30 [1962], there had been 332 cases of hearing damage attributed to high levels of noise in industrial plants.

These were reported in metal working plants where riveting was the chief offender; wood-working plants where saws made the noise; boiler plants, and in tunnel digging for building construction.

—Wallace Turner, "California Plans Noise Regulation," *The New York Times* (Western Edition), (January 15, 1963), pp. 9, 11.

That the average 70-to-79-year-old American has trouble understanding speech is a result not of aging *per se*. It is the result of his having lived so long in a world that has become noisier each year. The steadily intensified sonic attack on his ears has left him little to hear with.

—Berland, *The Fight for Quiet*, p. 11.

Hearing tests made on high school students in Tennessee suggest that the intensive, prolonged noise of discotheque rock music, played long and loud, actually kills some of the cells in the ears. The result: a boy of 17 may hear no better than a man of 65. This kind of damage is there for life.

—*Can Man Survive*, p. 6.

Rock and roll music has been measured at peaks of 122 dB in discothéques and teen dance halls . . . far above the 80 to 90 dB of noise which has long been established as the risk criterion level in industry.

—Still, *In Quest of Quiet*, p. 48.

The pain threshold is 120 dB for some ears. At 140, sound can be extremely painful, and 160-dB sound can kill small animals.

—Still, *In Quest of Quiet*, p. 54.

Persons who expose themselves to high-intensity rock music for a total exposure time exceeding twenty-three hours in a two-month period may suffer irreversible damage to the sensing cells in the ear [according to Dr. David M. Lipscomb, Director of Audiology Clinical Services at the University of Tennessee in Knoxville].

—Still, *In Quest of Quiet*, p. 53.

The deafness produced by noise is the result of the battering which the tiny hair cells in the cochlea receive. Microscopic studies of the inner ears of animals which were experimentally subjected to noise show how these cells swell and change shape. And the hair cells first affected are those closest to the oval window, which are responsible for sensing the higher frequencies heard. Apparently, if the noise stops soon enough

165

the hair cells suffer no permanent damage and repair themselves. Thus mended, they go on with their business of hearing. But if the noise doesn't stop soon enough, or if there isn't enough of a pause between noises to allow these cells to heal, they will stay permanently damaged and the noise-induced hearing loss will become permanent. Microscopic studies, again, show how the unrecovered cells simply disintegrate and disappear forever. If the noise is intense enough, and lasts long enough, and occurs frequently enough, the destruction of hair cells spreads and with it comes a spread in the frequencies that are lost to hearing. Depending on the nature of the noise exposure, all the working parts of the cochlea can be destroyed in time.

—Berland, *The Fight for Quiet,* p. 22.

. . . Samuel Rosen, M.D. of Mount Sinai Hospital and Columbia University, New York City . . . has led several teams of medical and hearing researchers into Sudan Africa . . . to study members of the Mabaan tribe, who are, as he has written, "a pre-Nilotic, pagan, primitive tribal people whose state of cultural development is the late Stone Age. They are a peaceful and quiet people, about 20,000 of them. . . ."

. . . He was amazed to see them converse 300 feet apart without raising their voices. "Hearing is significantly more acute in all Mabaans aged 10 through 70 years than in people of the same age who live in industrial areas of the United States. Except for the bleat of a goat and other sounds of nature, the Mabaans live in a dramatically quiet, almost silent atmosphere. The bombardment of excessive noise in our culture and the virtual absence of such in theirs could be one of the factors responsible for their superior hearing." He found that the average Mabaan man of 75 could hear as well as the average American man of 25.

—Berland, *The Fight for Quiet,* pp. 16–17.

In all fairness, I must say that absence of noise alone is not the only factor in preserving the fantastic hearing of the Mabaans. Dr. Rosen found another important factor: the ample blood supply to the ear, even in the aged. This . . . depends on the general health of the cardiovascular system, which itself relies on a host of factors, including diet, exercise, and heredity. One of these factors also is stress [,] and . . . noise adds a pertinent and dangerous stress on the body.

—Berland, *The Fight for Quiet*, p. 17.

Says Dr. Samuel Rosen, "Any loud noise, whether we like it or not, constricts blood vessels. Eventually, this could cause permanent damage." In addition to constricted vessels, says Dr. Rosen . . . there are other physiological reactions to noise: The skin pales, pupils dilate, eyes close and the voluntary and involuntary muscles tense. Gastric secretions diminish and adrenalin is suddenly injected into the blood stream. . . .

"If there is already present somatic disease like atherosclerosis or coronary heart disease, continued exposure to noise could endanger health and aggravate the pathology by adding insult to injury," Dr. Rosen suggests.

—Barbara J. Culliton, "Noise: Polluting the Environment," *Science News*, Vol. 97, No. 5 (January 31, 1970), p. 132.

All of the evidence points to the inescapable conclusion that the human cardiovascular system thrives in quiet, and that in modern civilized countries it reacts reflexly to the punishing noise that impinges upon it. Said [Dr. Gerd Jansen, a German research psychologist]: " . . . [Noise] is a stress applied to your body without your being aware of it. It can be, for instance, superimposed as an additional and subtle destructive factor on the diabetic's already impaired blood circulation."

—Berland, *The Fight for Quiet*, p. 98.

Odd as it may be to consider, noise even has its effects on the ears of the totally deaf. In 1958, U.S. Navy and Southwestern Medical School researchers tried loud noise (up to 170 dB) on ten such people. Starting at 120 dB, the five men and five women reported feeling vibration and tickles, and experiencing warmth, pain, and dizziness. Somehow, the researchers concluded, the loud noise had its effects on inner ear structures which also generally affected their bodies.

—Berland, *The Fight for Quiet*, p. 26.

Even machine noise so high in pitch we cannot hear it apparently affects not only our ears but our total health.

—Rienow and Rienow, p. 146.

Russian architect Constantin Stramentov, a specialist in noise control, wrote in the UNESCO *Courier* in its July, 1967 issue: . . . English radio audiences in 1966 heard Dr. John Anthony Parr say in an interview: One experiment conducted in France submitted a group of soldiers to a loud noise for 15 minutes. They were then tested and to everybody's surprise it was discovered they were color blind for over an hour.

—Berland, *The Fight for Quiet*, p. 105.

Like a drug that produces measurable effects when it enters the body, noise is being found to induce physiological changes that are suspected of having a relation to disease.

"Noise is a stress, an environmental pollutant, an insult," says Dr. Chauncey Leake of the University of California Medical Center at San Francisco. "It affects the nervous, endocrine and reproductive systems. It may damage unborn children."

—Culliton, "Noise-Polluting the Environment," *Science News* (January 31, 1970), p. 132.

According to Dr. Bruce Welch of the Friends of Psychiatric Research in Baltimore, "The physiological effects of sound are measurable at as low as 70 decibels. They are all-pervasive, most threatening to the young and yet difficult to spell out in man because problems arise from long-term, chronic exposure."

—Culliton, "Noise-Polluting the Environment," *Science News* (January 31, 1970), p. 132.

Noise, in experimental animals at least, also affects kidney function through its action on hormones. In 1964, Australian pharmacologist Dr. Mary F. Lockett was conducting tests on endocrine activity in rats when a violent thunderstorm occured in Perth. "The next morning," she recounts, "the animals were badly out of salt and water balance." Subsequently, she exposed the rats to recorded thunderclaps of 100 decibels at a low frequency of 150 cycles per second. The noise stimulated the release of a hormone, oxytocin, from the pituitary gland. Oxytocin, in turn, stimulated the kidney, resulting in enhanced excretion of salt and water. High-frequency sounds had another effect. They stimulated adrenalin secretion up to 20 times normal levels and caused water retention, rather than excretion, because adrenalin inhibits snythesis of antidiuretic hormone, which inhibits the excretion of fluids.

—Culliton, "Noise-Polluting the Environment," *Science News* (January 31, 1970), p. 132.

Dr. John L. Fuller of the Jackson Laboratories in Bar Harbor, Me., sees animals' response to noise as a valuable laboratory model for studying the biology of stress and the chemistry of the brain as it affects the nervous system. With Dr. Robert L. Collins, he has been looking at sound-induced seizures in inbred strains of mice. The genetic makeup of a mouse influences its response to noise. "Not all strains will convulse when stimulated by sound," Dr. Fuller explains, "but some are clearly more susceptible than others."

However, though genes play a role in this mouse syndrome, which has no exact counterpart in human medicine (except for rare cases of musicogenic epilepsy), Dr. Fuller has shown that environmental stress at the right time can convert a theoretically unsusceptible mouse into a convulsive one. If a mouse from a genetically resistant strain is subjected to loud sounds—95 decibels or more—on about the sixteenth day of life, subsequent noises will drive it into convulsions.

—Culliton, "Noise: Polluting the Environment," *Science News* (January 31, 1970), pp. 132–33.

Dr. Lester W. Sontag, Director of Fels Research Institute, Yellow Springs, Ohio, has studied the effects of noise on the human fetus. His experiments indicate that prenatal noise can cause predisposition to audiogenic seizures after birth. Citing this, and the results of other research as evidence, he believes that loud noises, and especially the sonic boom, can be as much a teratogen—an instigator of congenital malformations—as can such drugs as thalidomide and such viruses as German measles. Some of these effects of prenatal noise may be so

169

subtle as to be responsible decades later . . . [for] the behavior of the [adult] person. . . .

—Berland, *The Fight For Quiet*, p. 86.

In spite of the fact that researchers have yet to accumulate all of the data on the subject they would like, they agree it is reasonable to postulate that the greatest noise threat is to unborn and very young children. Presumably, the developing fetus, whose organs and tissues are taking form, is the most sensitive of biological systems. Sound constricting a mother's blood vessels could certainly take its toll on an unborn child.

—Culliton, "Noise-Polluting the Environment," *Science News* (January 31, 1970), p. 133.

While certain effects of noise can be observed in man, and while these effects can be more clearly defined in experimental animals in controlled circumstances, it is also apparent that in assessing its effects on man in relation to environmental disease, other factors, including genetics, the general health of the cardiovascular system and routine noise levels, must be considered.

—Culliton, "Noise: Polluting the Environment," *Science News* (January 31, 1970), p. 133.

Aircraft noises around London Airport, Heathrow, may cost £70 million a year, according to Dr E. J. Richards, vice-chancellor of Loughborough University and a former member of the Wilson committee on noise. This would be due to two factors: the rapid depreciation of house prices in the affected area, and the cost of people who could not stand the noise having to move to quieter places. Dr Richards arrives at the sum by the following argument. Houses within the disturbingly noisy area . . . lose their value [by] . . . depreciation . . . [at] an average annual loss of £50. . . . [The] number of houses . . . [brings the total] to £33 million. That represents the loss of house values within the noisy area. The other part of the sum covers the expenses of people who are seriously disturbed by the noise and have to pay the cost of moving. . . . Of course only a proportion of the two million people living within

170

the noise area . . . [will] move, but take the reasonable figure of 400,000 people, and assume that they move after three years. Assume, further, that the cost of moving . . . is £500, then the total "moving cost" is £33 million a year. Hence the overall sum is £66 million.

Richards admits that "This is obviously a rough shot, but basically it's right." He points out that there is no doubt of the benefit of Heathrow to the economy—to the tune of £300 million a year—but that no one has bothered to find out the "disbenefit" cost of the noise. . . .

. . . [Dr. Richards] believes that the gain in economic wealth to the community should be at least 100 times the cost of the nuisance caused, to justify going ahead [with proposed airport expansion]. It was true that aircraft manufacturers had made engines quieter, but the reductions they were able to make were "only playing at the game." . . .[The] nuisance value of [noise created at] Heathrow alone ran into millions; the sums [of money] to do something about it should also be in terms of millions.

—"Costing the Cacophony," New Scientist, Vol. 46, No. 700 (May 7, 1970), p. 269.

. . . James J. Harford, executive secretary of the American Institute of Aeronautics, writing on the Op-Ed page of this newspaper on Tuesday [December 1], offered some . . . breathtaking assertions. . . .

Mr. Harford asserts that the SST will cause "only" 2.5 pounds of "overpressure." But the Federal Government tactfully stopped sonic boom tests over Oklahoma City because overpressure of only 1.3 to 1.7 pounds provoked such painful noise levels. It is perfectly true that the SST will climb faster than the existing jumbo jets, but the harsh fact remains that while climbing from zero to 1,500 feet, the SST will make ear-shattering noise louder than anything today's jets produce. . . .

—"Downwind From the SST" (editorial), The New York Times (December 2, 1970), p. 46.

Noise destroyed the first generation of Comets [early British jetliners] by starting small cracks in the walls and making them grow until the metal failed. The next generation of jetliner may destroy our homes by starting small cracks and hitting them again and again until the walls fail. Thus does noise, in the form of the sonic boom especially, hang over our heads threatening to attack our health (both emotional and bodily), our hearing, and even our houses.

—Berland, *The Fight for Quiet*, p. 132.

8

DDT and Other Chemical Pollution

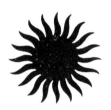

Organochlorine insecticides volatilize. When they are applied as sprays, and especially when they are applied as sprays from aircraft, they are likely to be widely dispersed in the atmosphere. They have been detected in both air and rainwater in Britain. At present large-scale aerial spraying operations are unusual in Europe. However, they are frequently carried out in order to combat forest pests in North America, and to control locusts in tropical countries; both operations may affect the amounts of pesticides falling on European countries.

—Norman Moore, "Pesticides Know no Frontiers," *New Scientist*, Vol. 46, No. 697 (April 16, 1970), pp. 114–115.

. . . Each year, more than 600 million pounds of pesticides of all kinds are sprayed, dusted, fogged, or dumped in the United States— about three pounds for every man, woman, and child in the country.

The residues drift through the air, mingle with the waters to destroy aquatic life, and seep through the soil to contaminate the environment on a worldwide basis. Pesticide particles have been found, for example, in the tissues of reindeer in Alaska, in penguins of the Antarctic, and in the dust over the Indian Ocean. Several species of animal life, including the American bald eagle, the peregrine falcon, the osprey, and the Bermuda petrel are on the verge of extinction by pesticides.

—Nelson, "Our Polluted Planet," *The Progressive* (November 1969), pp. 13–14.

The tissues of coastal wildlife in Antarctica harbor traces of pesticides that have never been used on the continent.

—"The Ravaged Environment," *Newsweek* (January 26, 1970), p. 31.

... [Living] organisms can themselves cause the dispersal of pesticides from one nation to another. Many species of fish and birds are migratory, and spend part of their lives in areas where pesticides are used extensively and migrate to others where they are not. . . . So there is some evidence that dispersal of pesticides by living organisms is having biological effects far from the treated areas.

—Moore, Pesticides Know no Frontiers," *New Scientist* (April 16, 1970), p. 115.

Louisiana's state bird, the brown pelican, has vanished from its shores (600 of the birds remain in an island colony off the California coast, but last year [1969] they produced only five chicks; the rest of their eggs collapsed with weakened shells that contained high concentrations of DDT).

—"The Ravaged Environment," *Newsweek* (January 26, 1970), p. 31.

Clearly residue levels that produce the "egg-shell thinning" effect are far below levels presumed to be safe by existing regulations. We may have to discard the entire "parts per million" approach. The problem of environmental consequences of widely distributed toxic residues is larger than we have thought.

—Robert L. Rudd, *Pesticides and the Living Landscape*, Madison, Wis.:University of Wisconsin Press, 1964, p. ix.

A two-year national pesticide study completed recently by the U.S. Bureau of Sport Fisheries and Wildlife found DDT in 584 of 590 samples of fish taken from forty-four rivers and lakes across the United States. The study revealed DDT residues ranging up to forty-five parts per million in the whole fish, a count more than *nine times higher* than the current Food and Drug Administration guideline level for DDT in fish.

—Nelson, "Our Polluted Planet," *The Progressive* (November 1969), p. 14.

The threat of pesticides to public health and safety was made shockingly obvious last spring [of 1969] when the Food and Drug Administration seized 28,000 pounds of pesticide-contaminated Coho salmon

176

in Lake Michigan. The concentration of DDT in the salmon was up to nineteen parts per million; the accumulation of dieldrin, a persistent and more toxic pesticide, up to 0.3 parts per million. Both levels are considered hazardous by the FDA and the World Health Organization.

—Nelson, "Our Polluted Planet," *The Progressive* (November 1969), p. 14.

In water, DDT may contaminate virtually all organisms *at all levels of the food chain.* Some examples:

—The Coho salmon accumulated residues in Lake Michigan and these were passed into the eggs. Recently almost 700,000 salmon fry died shortly after hatching.

—Heavy mortality of trout fry occured similarly in several New York lakes. For several years, mortality of fry from Lake George in New York was 100 percent.

—Wurster, "DDT-Danger to the Environment," *University Review* (Summer 1969), p. 25.

[According to the M.I.T.-sponsored "Study of Critical Environmental Problems," conducted in July 1970:] It is known that high levels of DDT residues are found in certain marine organisms; for instance, DDT residues in mackerel caught off the California coast exceed permissible tolerance levels for human consumption.

—Luther J. Carter, "The Global Environment: M.I.T. Study Looks for Danger Signs," *Science*, Vol. 169, No. 3946 (August 14, 1970), pp. 661–62.

BONN, June 25—A poisonous wave of insecticide washed out of West German waters today after killing millions of Rhine River fish and some ducks during the last six days. It is still lingering in the Netherlands, where about 100 tons of dead fish have washed up.

The source of the poison was identified by Dutch chemists last night as an insecticide called endosulfan and marketed as Thiodan (it is a sulphurous acid ester). . . .

German investigators . . . are working on the theory that either someone dumped more than 200 pounds of the poison in the river near

St. Goar or dusted the vineyards and fruit trees around St. Goar with endosulfan from the air last Wednesday and possibly again on Friday.

—David Binder, "Source of Fish Poisoning in Rhine Identified as Insecticide," *The New York Times* (June 26, 1969), p. 6.

PARIS, June 25—French conservationists charged today that insecticides such as the one that has polluted the Rhine River were responsible for deaths of people as well as wildlife.

They appealed to the new Minister of Agriculture, Jacques Duhamel, to impose a ban, held up, they said, in the Ministry for three years because of pressure from chemical companies.

Antoine Reille, a spokesman for the Federation of Societies for the Protection of Nature, said in an interview that world-wide conservation organizations were seeking an international agreement to halt pollution by organochlore insecticides. . . .

He angrily denied statements by West German officials Sunday that the insecticide in question was not harmful to human life.

Following an antimosquito campaign with similar chemicals in southwestern France, he said, an incomplete canvass of physicians disclosed 75 cases of poisoning of human beings, four of them fatal.

—"French Condemn Insecticides," *The New York Times* (June 26, 1969), p. 6.

The spillage in June 1969 of quantities of the organochlorine insecticide endosulfan into the River Rhine in Germany provides an example of gross contamination of water by a pesticide, and illustrates the international problems which ensue. Endosulfan is extremely toxic to fish: concentrations in the water as low as 0.00002 parts per million cause death. It was estimated that many million fish died in the Rhine as a result of the spillage. The Rhine and its tributaries flow through six countries, and pollution in one is liable to affect others. It is disturbing that eight months after the disaster no comprehensive report has yet been issued. It is urgently required in the interests of international cooperation in the control of pesticides in Europe.

—Moore, "Pesticides Know no Frontiers," *New Scientist* (April 16, 1970), p. 114.

River pollution can affect inshore coastal waters, which are the breeding grounds of fish of economic importance.

Pollution by spillage and effluents may be an important contributory source of global contamination. There is increasing evidence that in Britain, at any rate, industrial pesticide pollution is more important than pollution caused by run-off resulting from normal agricultural use. Some pollution is undoubtedly caused, though, by washing out spraying machinery and dumping used containers in water courses.

—Moore, "Pesticides Know no Frontiers," *New Scientist* (April 16, 1970), p. 114.

THE HAGUE, Feb. 21—Dutch scientists have concluded that polluted, dredged-up mud that was dumped offshore from Rotterdam was apparently responsible for the widespread deaths of a colony of seabirds a hundred miles away. . . .

The Dutch case came to light in 1964 and 1965, when numbers of fork-tailed birds known as sandwich terns were seen going into convulsions and dying. . . .

The dead terns were found near traces of pesticide manufactured at a plant just outside Rotterdam. The . . . [plant's] operator, Shell Nederland Chemie M.V., tightened up on its antipollution precautions and by 1966 the wave of unnatural deaths had stopped.

—Eric Pace, "Dutch Scientists Blame Polluted Dredged-Up Mud for Widespread Deaths of Seabirds 100 Miles Away," *The New York Times* (February 22, 1970), p. 4.

An irony of the whole pesticide saga is that, time and again, the bugs have come out on top. Hit the insects with a pesticide, and a few hardy generations later, adaptation has developed a new breed that is immune to it. Rather than seeking the obvious answer of an alternative pest control, our response has usually been to use greater doses of the same old ineffective stuff.

—Nelson, "Our Polluted Planet," *The Progressive* (November 1969), p. 14.

By adding just one alien component to a delicate balance, man sometimes triggers a series of dangerous changes. Nature immediately tries to restore the balance—and often overreacts. When farmers wipe out one pest with powerful chemicals, they may soon find their crops afflicted with pests that are resistant to the chemicals. Worse, the impact of a pesticide like DDT can be vastly magnified in food chains. Thus DDT kills insect-eating birds that normally control pests that now destroy the farmers' crops. The "domino theory" is clearly applicable to the environment.

—"Fighting to Save the Earth from Man," *Time* (February 2, 1970), p. 57.

Dangerous levels of DDT and other deadly pesticides have been found in tobacco and fruit, and vegetable producers constantly must take care to avoid having their crops banned from commercial markets.

—Nelson, "Our Polluted Planet," *The Progressive* (November 1969), p. 14.

[Since] . . . 1946, the use of synthetic pesticides has increased from a million pounds annually to the "massive dispersal" in 1965 of nearly *one billion* pounds. . . . [We] are at present ingesting eight times as much poison as we did in 1940, and by 1975 we will be absorbing four times as much as we are absorbing today [1966]. . . .

—Rienow and Rienow, *Moment in the Sun*, p. 133.

IS MOTHERS' MILK FIT FOR HUMAN CONSUMPTION?

Nobody knows. But if it were on the market it could be confiscated by the Food and Drug Administration. Why? Too Much DDT. We get it from the food we eat. It's in mothers' milk, and in the body of virtually every animal on Earth — including man. DDT kills birds and fish, interferes with their reproduction, decimates their populations. It causes cancer in laboratory test animals, and people killed by cancer carry more than twice as much DDT as the rest of us. Nobody knows for sure what DDT is doing to humans. But who wants to wait around to find out?

That's what this country is doing. Waiting. There's been a lot of talk, but little action. You heard DDT was banned. It wasn't. Those were just empty headlines. DDT is still being used, despite acceptable alternatives.

Intolerable? Of course. It is also illegal. . . . Two big federal agencies that are supposed to protect us are not doing their job. The Environmental Defense Fund has taken them to court to see that they do.

—Environmental Defense Fund, Advertisement in *The New York Times* (March 29, 1970), The Week in Review section, p. 6.

. . . An increasing number of nations has put partial or total restrictions on certain persistent organochlorine insecticides. . . .

. . .The obvious need . . . is for all nations to work together to overcome this [problem of pesticide contamination] and other environmental problems which affect all mankind.

—Moore, "Pesticides Know no Frontiers," *New Scientist* (April 16, 1970), p. 114.

A new generation of insecticides has been emerging in this country [the United States] with the gradual but steady decline in the use of persistent poisons like DDT. The substitute products are, for the most part, regarded as safer than the earlier types—but are the new poisons safe? . . .

One of the substitute products now under scrutiny is carbaryl (1-naphthyl-N-methylcarbamate), popularly known as Sevin. . . .

Carbaryl is . . . a broad-spectrum killer and thus destroys many beneficial organisms. This indiscriminate reduction of living matter can have serious effects on any ecosystem. In addition, there is great concern over reports that carbaryl is teratogenic (causes birth defects) in mammals.

—Ian C. T. Nisbet and Dallas Miner, "DDT Substitute," *Environment*, Vol. 13, No. 6 (July/August 1971), p. 10.

Last November [U.S.] Secretary [of Agriculture] Hardin "banned" . . .[the use of DDT] in residential areas, but the ban was immediately nullified by the slow-motion procedure on manufacturers' appeals. This order did not touch the Southern cotton fields where two-thirds of the DDT sold in this country is actually used. The Secretary has refused to suspend all use of DDT pending court review because he does not regard it as an "imminent hazard." Secretary Hardin insistently pleads for more evidence on issues that have already been abundantly researched. . . .

—"The Hardin Follies" (editorial), *The New York Times* (July 24, 1970), p. 30.

The World Health Organization has critically examined over 1000 . . . possible substitute pesticides to replace DDT in the worldwide antimalaria program, and has found none that can meet the essential requirements of availability, efficacy, safety, stability, and cost.

—Robert White-Stevens (Bureau of Conservation and Environmental Science, Rutgers University), in *Science*, Vol. 170, No. 3961 (November 27, 1970), p. 928.

. . .[Philip Handler's statement in *Science*, January 15, 1971], "The predicted death or blinding by parathion of dozens of Americans last summer must rest on the consciences of every car owner whose bumper sticker urged a total ban on DDT," is certainly nonsense unless he meant to add ". . . and also urged the present heavy use of organophosphates." Handler seems not to realize that the move to more toxic pesticides is due, not to bumper stickers, but to insect resistance to DDT. Insects live briefly and lay huge numbers of eggs, so they apparently will always become resistant to poisons before resistant strains of man can be selected. Is DDT now easy to ban because it does not kill most insect pests?

—Letter from Joe. L. Griffin, *Science*, Vol. 172, No. 3982 (April 30, 1971), pp. 425–26.

Between 1945 and 1963, the production of herbicides jumped from nine hundred and seventeen thousand pounds to about a hundred and seventeen thousand pounds in this country (the United States); since 1963, their use has risen two hundred and seventy-one per cent—more than double the rate of increase in the use of pesticides, though pesticides are still far more extensively used. By 1960, an area equivalent to more than three per cent of the entire United States was being sprayed each year with herbicides.

—Thomas Whiteside, *Defoliation*, (New York-Ballantine Books, 1970), pp. 5–6.

[Arthur W. Galston (professor of biology and lecturer in forestry, Yale University), speaking before the Subcommittee on National Security Policy and Scientific Developments of the Committee on Foreign Affairs of the House of Representatives, December 1969:]

"Since 1962, about 4 million acres of Vietnam have been sprayed with about 100 million pounds of assorted herbicides. This is an area about the size of the State of Massachusetts.

". . . The first type, Agent Orange, consists of two commonly used phenoxyacetic acids that go by the shorthand names of 2,4–D and 2,4,5–T.

"They are used in Vietnam at about 27 pounds per acre, and I should say parenthetically that this is up to ten times the usual domestic dose recommended."

—[Arthur W. Galston:] Whiteside, *Defoliation*, pp. 107–108.

"The kinds of undesirable consequences that flow from our massive use of herbicides can be summarized under three general headings. . . .

"One is ecological damage; the second would be inadvertent agricultural damage, and the third involves direct damage to people. . . .

"Up to a hundred thousand acres of these mangroves [lining the estuaries of Vietnam, especially around the Saigon River] have been sprayed. . . . Some of them had been sprayed as early as 1961, and have shown no substantial signs of recovery. . . .

". . . Ecologists have known for a long time that the mangroves lining the estuaries furnish one of the most important ecological niches for the completion of the life cycle of certain shellfish and migratory fish. If these plant communities are not in a healthy state, secondary effects on the whole interlocked web of organisms is bound to occur. . . . [In] the years ahead the Vietnamese, who do not have overabundant sources of protein anyhow, are probably going to suffer dietarily because of the deprivation of food in the form of fish and shellfish."

—Whiteside, *Defoliation*, pp. 109–10.

[Arthur W. Galston:]

"Damage to the soil is another possible consequence of extensive defoliation . . .

"We know that the soil is not a dead, inert mass, but, rather, that it is a vibrant, living community. . . . If you knock the leaves off of trees once, twice or three times, . . . you change the quality of the soil. . . .

". . . [Certain] tropical soils—and it has been estimated that in Vietnam up to 50 percent of all the soils fall into this category—are laterizable; that is, they may be irreversibly converted to rock as a result

183

of their deprivation of organic matter. . . . [If] you deprive trees of their leaves and photosynthesis stops, organic matter in the soil declines and laterization, the making of brick, may occur on a very extensive scale. I would emphasize that this brick is irreversibly hardened; it can't be made back into soil. . . ."

—Whiteside, *Defoliation*, pp. 110–11.

Picloram—whose use the Department of Agriculture has not authorized in the cultivation of any American crop—is one of the most persistent herbicides known. Dr. Arthur W. Galston . . . has described Picloram as "a herbicidal analog of DDT." . . . According to the authoritative "Merck Index," a source book on chemicals, this material is "poisonous." It can be used on agricultural crops in this country [the United States] only under certain restrictions imposed by the Department of Agriculture. It is being used herbicidally on Vietnamese rice fields at seven and a half times the concentration permitted for weed-killing purposes in this country, and so far in Vietnam something like five thousand tons is estimated to have been sprayed on paddies and vegetable fields.

—Whiteside, *Defoliation*, p. 7.

[Arthur W. Galston:]
"It is clear that picloram, once applied could be around for years. I would suggest that its massive application to the soils of Vietnam is going to hamper agriculture, even after hostilities are over, for some time into the future."

—Whiteside, *Defoliation*, p. 112.

[Arthur W. Galston:]
"My second category of damage is inadvertent agricultural damage. . . .

"We have documentation of several very important accidents of this kind in Vietnam. For example, thousands of trees in the Michelin rubber plantation to the north and west of Saigon were injured a few years ago following a spray operation. . . .

"In Cambodia we are now facing a lawsuit by the Cambodian Government to the extent of about $9 million resulting from extensive spraying in . . . neighboring South Vietnam. The report of the investigation team . . . concluded that only a part of the damage is due to inadvertent drift. Some damage appears to have been due to deliberate spraying over the Cambodian border. . . .

"There have been documented reports of extensive damage to truck crops along roads, trails, and canals near Saigon. . . . I believe the extent of this damage . . . certainly must go into the millions of dollars."

—Whiteside, *Defoliation*, pp. 112–13.

[Arthur W. Galston:] "Finally, I would like to discuss the most recent danger of the use of these herbicides to come to light. I refer to their direct damage to people. . . .

". . . It has recently been divulged that 2,4,5-T is one of the most teratogenic chemicals known. In experiments [on mice] by the Bionetics Laboratory in which 2,4,5-T was fed in the diet, in honey, from 4.6 up to 113 milligrams per kilogram [of] body weight, extensive teratogenic damage was noted. . . .

". . . At the highest concentration used, 113 milligrams . . ., which is equivalent to only a few ounces, for a human, 100 percent of all of the litters born had at least one abnormality, and up to 70 percent of all the offspring were abnormal in some major respect. . . .

"The results with mice were so striking that tests were conducted with rats, and the rat tests confirmed the teratogenicity. . . . "When the President's science advisor, Dr. DuBridge, was made aware of these results, he issued an order which restrained the use of 2,4,5-T, both domestically and in Vietnam. . . . In Vietnam, its use in populated areas is to be discontinued. The Department of Defense has announced that this is consistent with present use, and that operations involving 2,4,5-T will proceed as before.

"I suggest that its teratogenicity is such that even its use in such apparently innocuous domestic matters as clearing brush near powerlines is undesirable. Such chemicals could find their way into water supplies, and could be ingested in teratogenic doses. . . .

". . . [Significant] teratogenic events could have occurred among Vietnamese women. . . .

"If one looks at the Saigon newspapers, one finds that since late 1967, which would coincide with the end of the first year of our massive spray operations, there have been numerous reports . . . of the incidence

. . . of a completely new kind of birth abnormality. It is called the 'egg bundle-like fetus,' pictures of which have been published on the front pages of some of the Saigon newspapers.

"We do not know, of course, what is causing these abnormal births. There are many traumatic events occurring in South Vietnam. . . . But I would say that the entire spectrum of events compels me, as a biologist, to examine current restrictions on the use of all of these chemicals. . . . I would hope that further restrictions would be placed on the use of these chemicals. . . ."

—Whiteside, *Defoliation*, pp. 113–16.

Consider the case of the Herbicide 2,4,5-T. In 1968, after long study, a research laboratory under contract to the National Cancer Institute reported that 2,4,5-T produced birth defects when injected in mice and rats. Last October 29, Dr. Lee A. DuBridge, the President's science adviser, announced that the Department of Agriculture would cancel the use of 2,4,5-T on food crops after January 1, 1970 unless the Food and Drug Administration found a basis for establishing a safe legal tolerance.

The Food and Drug Administration found no such basis, but the New Year arrived with no action from Agriculture. Not until April did the department cancel the registrations authorizing the use of 2,4,5-T on lakes and ponds, in recreation areas and around homes. But no restriction was placed on its principal use—control of weeds on farms. Moreover, a survey of retail stores showed that it is still being sold to homeowners.

Five citizen organizations have been pressing [U.S.] Secretary [of Agriculture] Hardin to suspend any further use of this dangerous product. He has refused on grounds that it is not an "imminent hazard" to the public. The organizations have now petitioned in Federal Court in the District of Columbia for an order compelling him to act.

—"The Hardin Follies," *The New York Times* (July 24, 1970), p. 30.

. . . One team of investigators that considered the implications of human exposure to cadmium fifteen years ago glumly concluded: "Cadmium has probably more lethal possibilities than any of the other metals" [F.C. Christensen and E. C. Olsen, "Cadmium Poisoning,"

186

Archives of Industrial Health (Vol. 16, No. 8, 1957)]. Events since the group's report have borne out its assessment:

•Since 1962, officials of the Japanese ministry of Health and Welfare have registered 223 cases of severe degenerative bone disease attributed primarily to poisoning from cadmium mining wastes in one area of northern Japan [J. Kobayashi, "Relation Between Itai-Itai Disease and the Pollution of River Water by Cadmium from a Mine," presented at the 5th International Water Pollution Research Conference, July/August 1970]. . . .

•Some investigators find evidence that cadmium released into the environment is already taking a toll in lives in the United States. A statistical survey of 28 cities showed very good correlation between airborne cadmium and deaths caused by high blood pressure and arteriosclerotic heart disease [Robert E. Carroll, "The Relationship of Cadmium in the Air to Cardiovascular Disease Death Rates," *JAMA*, Vol. 198, No. 3 (October 17, 1966), pp. 267–69]. . . . General research to date indicates that cadmium in food and water in large concentrations may be a factor in hastening the aging process in human beings [Herbert E. Stokinger, "The Spectre of Today's Environmental Pollution —USA Brand: New Perspectives from an Old Scout," *American Industrial Hygiene Association Journal* (May–June 1969), pp. 195–217].

•There has been increased recognition of chronic poisoning to industrial workers who breathe in small amounts of cadmium compounds over an extended period of time [L. Friberg, "Chronic Cadmium Poisoning," *A.M.A. Archives of Industrial Health*, Vol. 20, (November 1959), pp. 401–407]. Primary effects are lung damage similar to pulmonary emphysema, kidney damage, and excessive urinary excretion of low molecular weight proteins. . . .

•The extent of environmental exposure is still uncertain, but recently completed information provides a rough measure of the situation in the United States:

•An estimated 4.6 million pounds of cadmium in various compounds are emitted into the atmosphere each year from a wide variety of cadmium processing and manufacturing activities and from the use and disposal of many commercial cadmium-containing products ranging from rubber tires to colored plastic bottles [*National Inventory of Sources and Emissions—Cadmium, Nickel, and Asbestos, 1968*, Cadmium, Section I, W. E. Davis & Associates, Environmental Protection

187

Agency, National Air Pollution Control Administration (Durham, N.C., February 1970)].

•Cadmium was detected in 42 percent of some 720 samples from rivers and reservoirs in the United States in 1970 [*Reconnaissance of Selected Minor Elements in Surface Waters of the United States—October 1970,* Geological Survey Circular 643, U.S. Geological Survey (Washington, D.C.)]. About 4 percent of the samples had levels of cadmium that exceeded the mandatory U.S. Public Health Service limit for drinking water. . . .

•Human beings take in significant quantities of cadmium compounds in food and beverages. Some of the cadmium is of natural origin, but much is introduced by man's activities. Cadmium-containing fertilizers and pesticides are a major source. These products contaminate soil and water, and the metal finds its way into certain crops, meat, fish, and tobacco [Henry A. Schroeder, et al., "Essential Trace Metals in Man: Zinc. Relation to Environmental Cadmium," *Journal of Chronic Diseases,* Vol. 20, pp. 179–210 (April 1967)]. Intake in food levels varies with a person's eating habits and may reach high levels.

•Americans take in amounts of cadmium in air, water, food, beverages, and cigarettes; the cadmium accumulates in the body in concentrations far greater than those which have caused biochemical liver changes, high mortality, and shortened life span in experimental animals [Robert Nilsson, "Aspects on the Toxicity of Cadmium and its Compounds," *Ecological Research Committee Bulletin No. 7,* Natural Science Research Council, Stockholm, Sweden].

—Julian McCaull, "Building a Shorter Life," *Environment,* Vol. 13, No, 7 (September 1971), pp. 3–4.

There are no cadmium ores, as such, as the metal is produced as a by-product in refining other metals, primarily zinc. Cadmium resembles zinc in chemical properties and is so closely associated with it in ores that the very name cadmium derives from the word calamine, a natural zinc compound. A certain amount of cadmium is in most multiple-metallic ore, however. . . . Cadmium dust, fumes, and mist are common by-products during refining of zinc, copper, and lead, as well as during extraction of cadmium.

—McCaull, "Building a Shorter Life," *Environment* (September 1971), p. 4.

188

. . . [One] source of cadmium wastes is the nickel-cadmium battery industry. . . . One [battery-making] plant on a stream that fed into the Hudson River discharged so much cadmium-containing waste that mud from the stream was 16.2 percent cadmium and 22.6 percent nickel by dry weight before state authorities cracked down, according to Dr. Henry A. Schroeder of Dartmouth Medical School. "It is a good place to mine cadmium," Dr. Schroeder observed.

—McCaull, *Environment* (September 1971), p. 7.

Widespread incidents of methyl-mercury poisoning have been reported only in recent decades. In Japan, more than 168 illnesses and 52 deaths were reported in two separate incidents in the 1950's from consumption of mercury-contaminated fish. Since 1960, more than 450 persons in several countries have become seriously ill and many have died from eating seed grain that had been treated with mercury compounds. Recently three children in New Mexico sustained severe brain damage after having eaten pork from animals that had been fed treated seed grain.

—Allen L. Hammond, "Mercury in the Environment," *Science*, Vol. 171, No. 3973 (February 26, 1971), p. 788.

The largest uses of mercury at present are for the electrolytic production of chlorine and caustic soda and for the manufacture of electrical equipment and antifouling paint. Substantial amounts are also consumed in agriculture as pesticides and seed treatments. Consumption of the metal in the United States since 1900 has been about 10^5 [one million] metric tons, with world consumption probably several times as great. Reliable estimates of how much of this has been lost to the environment are hard to come by, but it may be as much as a third. World production of mercury is currently about 9000 metric tons a year. Discharges from industrial plants into rivers, incineration of used electrical equipment, exhausts from metal smelters, and crop applications put mercury into the air, soil, and waterways.

In addition to losses from direct uses, mercury is released in the combustion of coal and petroleum products. The mercury content of these fuels varies widely, depending on their source. . . . Really systematic studies have yet to be done, but a number of investigators report concentrations averaging 1 ppm [part per million] in coal.

—Hammond, "Mercury in the Environment," *Science* (February 26, 1971), p. 789.

While mercury is known to be present in most foods, attention has focused on fish where mercury levels have been the highest. It is now known that the greatest mercury concentrations are found in older predatory fish. . . .

. . . The closer the fish is to the top of the food chain, the more mercury it will have taken in from its prey farther down the chain.

Tuna and swordfish, both large, predatory fish, accumulate mercury for years before reaching a commercially valuable size.

To some degree, fish and animals have always been accumulating mercury. Now, it appears, man's extraction of mercury from ore and eventual disposal of it into streams and lakes and, eventually, into the oceans may be increasing the amount to be taken into the food chain.

Many industries once thought disposal of metallic mercury in the water was safe because metallic mercury itself is not especially harmful. It was known that the danger lay in organic compounds of mercury.

Subsequently, it was found that certain microorganisms living in bottom muds can convert metallic mercury to an organic form called methyl mercury—the most toxic form.

—Boyce Rensberger, "Mercury and Man: A Puzzle for Ecologists," *The New York Times* (May 21, 1971), p. 30.

Man's use of mercury needs to be especially cautious, because, unlike some other pollutants, the difference between the tolerable natural background levels in the environment and levels harmful to man and animals is very small, and this may also turn out to be true for other heavy metals.

—Hammond, "Mercury in the Environment," *Science* (February 26, 1971), p. 789.

Over the last 20 years, . . . there has been a large increase in use of mercury compounds, both in industry (as catalysts in the manufacture of various plastics) and in agriculture (organomercury fungicides have greatly improved germination success in cereal crops). Both have resulted in extensive contamination of the environment: in the United

States, for example, waste containing 2000 tons of mercury is discharged into the environment annually.

. . . In Sweden (with a discharge rate of 70 tons pa [per annum] the effect [of mercury] on the ecosystem is receiving careful study. This followed alarm at the disappearance of the seed-eating Yellow Bunting from farmland areas using organomercury seed dressings. High levels of contamination were found in streams, and those in which levels exceeded one part per million were closed to fishermen. In 1966 the use of seed dressings was restricted, and since then the levels in the terrestrial ecosystem have fallen significantly (with the return of the buntings). However, even four years later, the level in the aquatic ecosystem is still rising as a legacy of accumulations is gradually leached out of the ground. It is thought that at least another 50 years are required to flush the whole ecosystem. Meanwhile at the top of the food chain, the grebes and ospreys continue to accumulate high levels in their bodies. The consequences of this cannot be predicted.

—"Mercury in the Environment," *New Scientist*, Vol. 47, No. 711 (July 23, 1970), p. 172.

Mercury is an insidious poison. Dr. Alan Hinsman, of the Viral Diseases Branch of the Center for Disease Control told a *New York Times* writer that with each exposure to mercury, damage to tissues may accumulate, even if the poison itself does not stay in the body. "Only one brain cell at a time may be killed," Dr. Hinsman said, "but eventually they add up. By the time you notice the effect, it's too late."

—Small, *Third Pollution*, p. 45.

Then there is the case of the mercury fungicide. Three children in New Mexico became gravely ill last February [1969] when they ate meat from a hog which had been fed seed treated with a mercury fungicide. The Agriculture Department with considerable publicity publicly banned further sale of this fungicide. But when one manufacturer refused to recall stocks already in the hands of distributors, the department quietly permitted continued sale of existing supplies. This contrasts sharply with Interior Secretary Hickel's attitude in asking for Government prosecution of companies polluting lakes and rivers with mercury. . . .

—"The Hardin Follies," *The New York Times* (July 24, 1970), p. 30.

When some Japanese mothers shrieked the Japanese equivalent of "Ouch, Ouch" after World War II, physicians did not know what caused their bones to pain so severely.

Only recently did doctors learn that these mothers' pains were caused by chronic cadmium poisoning. Few Americans are familiar with this disease that the Japanese call "Itai, Itai"—"Ouch, Ouch." . . .

"Itai, Itai" killed about 50 per cent of its more than 200 victims among the 24,000 Japanese who lived along a stream of the Jintsu River in Fuchu-machi in Toyama Prefecture. . . .

A cadmium mining plant upstream from the Fuchu-machi farming community, Dr. Kenza-buro Tsuchiya reported in the *Kelo Journal of Medicine* last year, had discharged its metal wastes into a river that deposited cadmium particles in its rice paddies.

Japanese absorbed the cadmium from the contaminated food and water they ate. The accumulated cadmium damaged their bodies and produced symptoms of "Itai, Itai." As evidence, . . . investigators reported high cadmium concentrations in rice and soybeans grown in the area.

In this country, cadmium poisoning is a rarely diagnosed industrial hazard. It chiefly affects welders, smelters and other metallurgic workers exposed to cadmium in plating processes.

When these workers inhale its fumes, cadmium can produce a severe lung inflammation producing chest pain, cough and difficult breathing. Inhalation cadmium poisoning kills one in five victims. . . .

Doctors have studied environmental cadmium in this country. In The Journal of the American Medical Association four years ago [1966], Dr. Robert E. Carroll reported that the average concentration of cadmium in the air of 28 American cities showed a marked correlation with death rates from high blood pressure and arteriosclerotic heart disease.

Other doctors have reported that patients with high blood pressure had increased cadmium levels in their kidneys. Still others believe cadmium pollution is a major factor in producing high blood pressure, which affects 23 million Americans.

—Lawrence K. Altman, "Japanese Diagnose Cadmium Disease," *The New York Times* (November 22, 1970), p. 73.

9

SST Pollution

The supersonic transport will fly at 60,000 ft., where there is no atmospheric turbulence or weather to bring pollutants down to earth. Even assuming that the plane has a fumeless engine, the water vapor in its exhaust may accumulate in the stratosphere, reflecting sunlight away from the earth.

—"Fighting to Save the Earth from Man," *Time* (February 2, 1970), p. 61.

An M.I.T.-sponsored "Study of Critical Environmental Problems" conducted on the Williams College Campus last month [July 1970] by some of the nation's most eminent environmental scientists . . . expressed "genuine concern" about the possibility that a large SST fleet might cause increased stratospheric cloudiness. . . . [The group] said that the SST's may cause water vapor in the atmosphere to increase by 10 percent globally, or by as much as 60 percent over the North Atlantic, where the SST traffic is expected to be heaviest.

Moreover, the group raised a possibility apparently never considered heretofore in the SST debate—that the [projected] SST fleet [of 500 SST's], by discharging combustion products such as soot, hydrocarbons, nitrogen oxides, and sulfate particles, would cause stratospheric smog, a condition that might also be especially pronounced over the North Atlantic. The group . . . by no means ruled out the possibility of stratospheric smogging causing temperature changes in the lower atmosphere and the earth's surface.

—Carter, "The Global Environment," *Science* (August 14, 1970), pp. 660–61.

... [The] SST would cost at least twice as much as the 747 and would consume twice as much fuel while carrying only two-thirds as many passengers. It could only be commercially viable if passengers were willing to pay a stiff surcharge for flying in it. . . .

—"Downwind From the SST," *The New York Times* (December 2, 1970), p. 46.

[According to] . . . Henry C. Wallich, professor of economics at Yale University, member of the Council of Economic Advisers in 1959–60, and currently chief consultant to the Secretary of the U.S. Treasury [:] "If it were possible to outlaw supersonic transport, no matter what countries would build and operate them, a strong case could be made for pronouncing such a ban. The gains from faster and more frequent travel seem small, relative to the injury from noise and possibly other environmental damage. Unfortunately, this decision is not in our hands. The Concorde is being built and will fly, whether or not the SST is built."

—John Lear, "Teaching in the Big School," *Saturday Review* (January 2, 1971), p. 66.

. . . To prevent sonic boom over land, the SST must fly subsonically over land, and the plane's operating efficiency goes down by at least 20 per cent. With airlines already losing money in the jumbo 747s, can they survive even more expense?

—John Lear, "Teaching in the Big School," *Saturday Review* (January 2, 1971), p. 66.

In the words of famed physicist Max Born, who died in 1970 at age eighty-seven, "Intellect distinguishes between the possible and the impossible; reason distinguishes between the sensible and the senseless. Even the possible can be senseless."

There is little doubt that the supersonic transport is possible. Time will tell if it is senseless.

—Still, *In Quest of Quiet*, p. 133.

196

. . . Senator William Proxmire, foe of superfluous spending and the SST, was particularly incensed when he came across an outlay by the [U.S.] Transportation Department, for $12,872. The funds were spent for publication of a children's book entitled "The Supersonic Pussycat." . . .

—"Spectrum," *Environment* (September, 1971), p. 28.

[U Thant (then U.N. Secretary general), May 11, 1971:] "I believe that mankind is at last aware of the fact that there is a delicate equilibrium of physical and biological phenomena on and around the earth which cannot be thoughtlessly disturbed as we race along the road of technological development . . . This global concern in the face of a grave common danger, which carries the seeds of extinction for the human species, may well prove to be the elusive force which can bind men together. The battle for human survival can only be won by all nations joining together in a concerted drive to preserve life on this planet."

—UNESCO Courier.

Sources Cited

＊

ACKNOWLEDGMENTS

The publisher and compiler acknowledge with appreciation the permissions granted by the following copyright holders and others for the reprinted excerpts used in this book:

Air Pollution Control Association
Kurker, Charles, "Reducing Emissions from Refuse Disposal." *Journal of the Air Pollution Control Association*, Vol. 19, No. 2 (Feb. 1969), pp. 69–72.
Larsen, Ralph I., "Relating Air Pollution Effects to Concentration and Control." *Journal of the Air Pollution Control Association*, Vol. 20, No. 4 (April 1970), pp. 214–225.

American Chemical Society
Chow, Tsaihwa, and Earl, John L., "Trend of Increasing Lead Aerosols in the Atmosphere." Paper delivered at the annual meeting of the American Chemical Society, Feb. 25, 1970.
Kenahan, Charles B., "Solid Waste—Resources out of Place." *Environmental Science and Technology*, Vol. 5, No. 7 (July 1971), pp. 594–600. Copyright 1971 by the American Chemical Society.
Knapp, Carol E., "Recycling Sewage Biologically." *Environmental Science and Technology*, Vol. 5, No. 2 (Feb. 1971), pp. 112–113, Copyright 1971 by the American Chemical Society.
Mallin, H. Martin, Jr., "Utility Concept of Solid Waste Handling Makes Gains." *Environmental Science and Technology*, Vol. 5, No. 9 (Sept. 1971), pp. 752–753. Copyright 1971 by the American Chemical Society.
Miller, Stanton S., "A Solid Waste Recovery System for all Municipalities." *Environmental Science and Technology*, Vol. 5, No. 2 (Feb. 1971), pp. 109–111. Copyright 1971 by the American Chemical Society.

Christian Science Monitor
Dillin, Jack, "Researchers Wrestle with Challenge of City Noise." *Christian Science Monitor*, Sept. 13, 1965, p. 13 © 1965 The Christian Science Publishing Society. All rights reserved.

Journal of the American Medical Association (JAMA)

Albright, Edwin C., and Allday, Robert W., "Thyroid Carcinoma after Radiation Therapy for Adolescent Acne Vulgaris," *JAMA*, Vol. 199, No. 4 (January 23, 1967), pp. 280–281.

Conrad, Robert A., and Hicking, Arobati, Abstract of "Medical Findings in Marshallese People Exposed to Fallout Radiation." *JAMA*, Vol. 192, No. 6 (May 10, 1965).

Rosenthal, David S., and Beering, Steven C., "Hypogonadism after Microwave Radiation." *JAMA*, Vol. 205, No. 4 (July 22, 1968), pp. 245–248.

Simon, Norman, and Harley, John, "Skin Reactions from Gold Jewelry Contaminated with Radon Deposit." *JAMA*, Vol. 200, No. 3 (April 17, 1967), pp. 254–255.

Zaret, Milton M. Letter. *JAMA*, Vol. 217, No. 4 (July 26, 1971), p. 481.

"Control of Noises." *JAMA*, Vol. 213, No. 11 (Sept. 14, 1970), p. 1771. Reprint from *JAMA*, Sept. 14, 1895.

"Environmental Quality—Its Significance in Our Society." Editorial, *JAMA*, Vol. 213, No. 11 (Sept. 14, 1970), pp. 1890–1892.

"Irradiation in Utero." Editorial, *JAMA*, Vol. 192, No. 5 (May 3, 1965), p. 410.

"The Price of Automobiles." *JAMA*, Vol. 213, No. 9 (Aug. 31, 1970), p. 1419.

"The Role of Air Pollution in Chronic Obstructive Pulmonary Disease." *JAMA*, Vol. 214, No. 5 (Nov. 2, 1970), pp. 894–899.

"What Standards for Air Quality?" *JAMA*, Vol. 214, No. 9 (Nov. 30, 1970), p. 1717.

The Lancet

Stewart, Alice, and Kneale, G. W., "Radiation Dose Effects in Relation to Obstetric X-Rays and Childhood Cancers." *The Lancet*, June 6, 1970, p. 1185.

"X-Rays and Childhood Cancer." Editorial, *The Lancet*, March 16, 1968, pp. 577–578.

Los Angeles Times

Reston, Richard, "British Experts Warn Pollution Perils Life." *Los Angeles Times*, February 24, 1971, p. 26. Copyright, 1971, Los Angeles Times.

Microforms International Marketing Corp.

Murozumi, M., Chow, Tsaihwa, J., AND Patterson, C., "Chemical Concentrations of Pollutant Lead Aerosols, Terrestrial Dusts and Sea Salts in the Greenland and Antarctic Snow Strata." *Geochimica et Cosmo chimica Acta* Vol. 33 (1969), pp. 1247–1294.

National Center for Air Pollution Control
for the following material from the Proceedings of the Third National Conference on Air Pollution. Public Health Service Publication No. 169 *(COAP)*.
Fuller, Louis J., "Concluding Remarks." *COAP*, pp. 458–459.
Moore, William W., "Radiation in Ambient Air Concentration of Fly Ash —Present and Future Prospects." *Coap*, pp. 170–178.
Nelson, Gaylord, "A Congressional View of the Problem." *COAP*, pp. 450–53.
Ryan, William F., "A Congressional View of the Problem." *COAP*, pp. 342–347.
Smith, Maynard E., "Reduction of Ambient Air Concentrations of Pollutants by Dispersion from High Stacks." *COAP*, pp. 151–160.
Sporn, Philip, "Discussion of Preceding Three Papers." *COAP*, pp. 143–147.
Udall, Stewart L., "Development of National Policy with Respect to Coal and Oil." *COAP*, pp. 128–130.

National Parks and Conservation Magazine
(which assumes no responsibility for distribution of the following article other than through this magazine):
Hechler, Ken, "TVA Ravages the Land." *National Parks and Conservation Magazine*, Vol. 45, No. 7 (July 1971), pp. 15–16.

National Tuberculosis and Respiratory Disease Association
Air Pollution Primer. New York: National Tuberculosis and Respiratory Disease Association, 1969.

Natural History
Winn, Ira J., "Greetings from Los Angeles." *Natural History*, Vol. 80, No. 8 (Oct. 1971), pp. 16, 18. Copyright © 1971 by the American Museum of Natural History.

Newark, N.J., *Evening News*
Staples, James M., "Lead Particles in Air Seen as Peril to Brain, Blood and Bones." *The* (Newark, N.J.) *Evening News*, April 29, 1971, p. 26.

New Scientist
The following appeared first in *New Scientist*, the weekly review of science and technology, 128 Long Acre, London WC 2:
Harris, A. L., Letter. *New Scientist*, Vol. 46, No. 700 (May, 1970), pp. 300–301.
Moore, Norman, "Pesticides Know No Frontiers." *New Scientist*, Vol. 46, No. 697 (April 16, 1970), pp. 114–115.

"Costing the Cacophony." *New Scientist,* Vol. 46, No. 700 (May, 1970), p. 269.

"Mercury in the Environment." *New Scientist,* Vol. 47, No. 711 (July 23, 1970), p. 172.

Newsweek
"The Ravaged Environment." *Newsweek,* Jan. 26, 1970, pp. 31–39. Copyright Newsweek, Inc. 1970.

New York Board of Trade
The Mayor's Task Force on Noise Control, *Toward a Quieter City.* New York: New York Board of Trade, 1970.

The New York Times
Altman, Lawrence K., "Japanese Diagnose Cadmium Disease." *The New York Times,* Nov. 22, 1970, p. 73. © 1970 by The New York Times Company.

Binder, David, "Source of Fish Poisoning in Rhine Identified as Insecticide." *The New York Times,* June 26, 1969, p. 6. © 1969 by The New York Times Company.

Bird, David, "Risk in Dirt Particles Found in City's Air." *The New York Times,* Sept. 20, 1971, p. 51. © 1971 by The New York Times Company.

Faust, Joan Lee, ". . . But Air Pollution Threatens." *The New York Times,* October 25, 1970, p. 39, Arts & Leisure section, © 1970 by The New York Times Company.

Gitlin, David, M.D., Letter. *The New York Times.* Nov. 15, 1970, p. 10, The Week in Review section. © 1970 by The New York Times Company.

Hill, Gladwin, "Purification of Nation's Waters Expected to Be Long and Costly." *The New York Times,* March 17, 1970, pp. 1, 29. © 1970 by The New York Times Company.

Hill, Gladwin, "Statistics Can Becloud the Pollution Picture." *The New York Times,* Dec. 28, 1970, p. 26. © 1970 by The New York Times Company.

Hill, Gladwin, "Texas Pollution Spurs Action by U.S." *The New York Times,* Jan. 19, 1970, p. 33. © 1970 by The New York Times Company.

Hofmann, Paul, "After a Century as Italy's Capital, the Eternal City Suffers Modern Agonies." *The New York Times,* Sept. 21, 1970. © 1970 by The New York Times Company.

Kenworthy, E. W., "The Airlines Accept Pollution Deadline." *The New York Times,* Jan. 21, 1970, pp. 1, 26. © 1970 by The New York Times Company.

Lyons, Richard D., "Return to Detergents with Phosphates Urged by Government in Shift of Policy." *The New York Times,* Sept. 16, 1971, pp. 1, 37 © 1971 by The New York Times Company.

Macdonald, Ross, and Easton, Robert, "Santa Barbarans Cite an 11th Com-

mandment: Thou Shalt Not Abuse the Earth." *The New York Times Magazine*, Oct. 12, 1969, pp. 32–33. © 1969 by The New York Times Company.
Pace, Eric, "Dutch Scientists Blame Polluted Dredged-up Mud for Widespread Death of Seabirds 100 Miles Away." *The New York Times*, Feb. 22, 1970, p. 4. © 1970 by The New York Times Company.
Rensberger, Boyce, "Mercury and Man: A Puzzle for Ecologists." *The New York Times*, May 21, 1971, p. 30. © 1971 by The New York Times Company.
Ripley, Anthony, "Infants and Radioactive Sands: Small-Town Doctor Wins Fight." *The New York Times*, Oct. 3, 1971, p. 75. © 1971 by The New York Times Company.
Ripley, Anthony, "Radioactive Building Sand Stirs Dispute." *The New York Times*, Sept. 27, 1971, pp. 1, 15. © 1971 by The New York Times Company.
Ripley, Anthony, "Radioactive Sands Linked to Higher Death Rates," *The New York Times*, Oct. 28, 1971, p. 27. © 1971 by The New York Times Company.
Seaborg, Glenn, "Do We Need Nuclear Power?" *The New York Times*, Dec. 28, 1970, p. 31. © 1970 by The New York Times Company.
Schmeck, Harold M., Jr., "Caution on X-Ray: Don't Overdo It." *The New York Times*, Oct. 15, 1967, p. 6, The Week in Review section. © 1967 by The New York Times Company.
Schmeck, Harold M., Jr., "Scientist Links Mediocrity to Fetuses Damaged in Lax X-Ray Examinations." *The New York Times*, Oct. 12, 1967, p. 35. © 1967 by The New York Times Company.
Semple, Robert B., "Great Lakes Pact Signed in Ottawa by Nixon, Trudeau." *The New York Times*, April 16, 1972, pp. 1, 3. © 1972 by The New York Times Company.
Sullivan, Walter, "Oil Called Peril to Food Supply in Sea." *The New York Times*, Jan. 16, 1970, p. 18. © 1970 by The New York Times Company.
Turner, Wallace, "California Plans Noise Regulation." *The New York Times* (Western Edition), Jan. 15, 1963, pp. 9, 11. © 1963 by The New York Times Company.
Wilcke, Gerd, "Detergent Companies Hail U.S. Step on Phosphates." *The New York Times*, Sept. 16, 1971, p. 37. © 1971 by The New York Times Company.
"Downwind from the SST." Editorial, *The New York Times*, Dec. 2, 1970, p. 46. © 1970 by The New York Times Company.
"French Condemn Insecticides." *The New York Times*, June 26, 1969, p. 6. © 1969 by The New York Times Company.
"The Hardin Follies." Editorial, *The New York Times*, July 24, 1970, p. 30. © 1970 by The New York Times Company.

"Lead Is Studied in Coastal Fish." *The New York Times,* Dec. 27, 1970, p. 23. © 1970 by The New York Times Company.

"Swiss Scientist Estimates Seas Will Die in 25 Years." *The New York Times,* Oct. 26, 1971, p. 5. © 1971 by The New York Times Company.

"Trouble on Oily Waters." Editorial, *The New York Times,* July 19, 1970, p. 12, The Week in Review section. © 1970 by The New York Times Company.

"Whitewash for Phosphates." Editorial, *The New York Times,* Sept. 22, 1971, p. 46. © 1971 by The New York Times Company.

W. W. Norton & Company, Inc.
Benarde, Melvin A., *Our Precarious Habitat.* New York: Norton, 1970, pp. 155, 165. Copyright © 1970 by W. W. Norton & Company, Inc.
Carr, Donald E., *Death of the Sweet Waters.* New York: Norton, 1966, pp. 47, 69, 145, 148, 151, 152. Copyright © 1966 by W. W. Norton & Company, Inc.

Popular Science Publishing Co., Inc.
Fisher, Arthur, "Science Newsfront." *Popular Science,* Oct. 1971.

Praeger Publishers, Inc.
Small, William E., *Third Pollution: The National Problem of Solid Waste Disposal.* New York: Praeger, 1971. © 1971 by Praeger Publishers, Inc., New York.

Prentice-Hall, Inc.
Berland, Theodore, *The Fight for Quiet.* Englewood Cliffs, N.J.: Prentice-Hall, 1970. © 1970 by Theodore Berland.

The Progressive
Nelson, Gaylord A., "Our Polluted Planet." *The Progressive,* Vol. 33, No. 11 (Nov. 1969), pp. 13–17.

G. P. Putnam's Sons
Montagu, Ashley, *The American Way of Life.* New York: Putnam, 1967. Copyright © 1952, 1962, 1967 by Ashley Montagu. Adapted for this book by the author.

Radiological Society of North America
Webster, Edward W., "Hazards of Diagnostic Radiology: A Physicist's Point of View." *Radiology,* Vol. 72, No. 4 (April, 1959), p. 498.

Ramparts
Gellen, Martin, "The Making of a Pollution-Industrial Complex." *Ramparts,* Vol. 8, No. 11 (May 1970), pp. 23, 24.
Rapoport, Roger, "Catch 24,400 (or, Plutonium Is My Favorite Element)." *Ramparts,* Vol. 8, No. 11 (May 1970), pp. 16–21.

Resources for the Future, Inc.
Headley, J. C., and Lewis, J. N., *The Pesticide Problem: An Economic Approach to Public Policy.* Washington, D. C.: Resources for the Future, Inc., 1967.

Saturday Review
Lear, John, "Teaching in the Big School." *Saturday Review,* Jan, 2, 1971, pp. 63–66. Copyright 1971 Saturday Review, Inc. By permission of the publisher and the author.
Lindsay, Sally, ed., "Earth Watch." *Saturday Review,* Nov. 7, 1970, p. 70. Copyright 1970 Saturday Review, Inc. By permission of the publisher and the author.
Schaeffer, John R., "Reviving the Great Lakes." *Saturday* Review, Nov. 7, 1970, pp. 63–65. Copyright 1970 Saturday Review, Inc. By permission of the publisher and the author.

Science, Published by the American Association for the Advancement of Science (AAAS)
Abelson, Philip H., "Marine Pollution." *Science,* Vol. 171, No. 3966 (Jan. 8, 1971), p. 21. Copyright 1971 by the AAAS.
Abelson, Philip H., "Excessive Emotion About Detergents." *Science,* Vol. 169, No. 3950 (Sept. 11, 1970), p. 1033. Copyright 1970 by the AAAS.
Carter, Luther J., "The Global Environment—M.I.T. Study Looks for Danger Signs." *Science,* Vol. 169, No. 3946 (Aug. 14, 1970), pp. 660–662. Copyright 1970 by the AAAS.
Chase, Grafton D., and Osol, Arthur, Letter. *Science,* Vol. 128, No. 3327 (Oct. 3, 1958), p. 788.
Eisenbud, Merril, "Environmental Protection in the City of New York." *Science,* Vol. 170, No. 3959 (Nov. 13, 1970), p. 706–712. Copyright 1970 by the AAAS.
Griffin, Joe L., Letter. *Science,* Vol. 172, No. 3982 (April 30, 1971), pp. 425–426. Copyright 1971 by the AAAS.
Hammond, Allen L., "Mercury in the Environment." *Science,* Vol. 171, No. 3973 (Feb. 26, 1971), pp. 788–789. Copyright 1971 by the AAAS.
Holden, Constance, "Nader Group Sees 'Water Wasteland.' " *Science,* Vol. 172, No. 3982 (April 30, 1971), pp. 455. Copyright 1971 by the AAAS.
Landsberg, Helmut E., "Man-Made Climatic Changes." *Science,* Vol. 170, No. 3964 (Dec. 18, 1970), pp. 1265–1274. Copyright 1970 by the AAAS.
Lave, Lester B., and Seskin, Eugene P., "Air Pollution and Human Health." *Science,* Vol. 169, No. 3947 (Aug. 21, 1970), pp. 723–733. Copyright 1970 by the AAAS.
Marx, Leo, "American Institutions and Ecological Ideals." *Science,* Vol. 170,

No. 3951 (Nov. 27, 1970), pp. 945–952. Copyright 1970 by the AAAS.
Morgan, George B., Ozolins, Gontis, and Tabor, Elbert C., "Air Pollution Surveillance Systems." *Science*, Vol. 170, No. 3955 (Oct. 16, 1970), pp. 289–296. Copyright 1970 by the AAAS.
Nelson, Bryce, "Hiroshima after 25 Years: 'We Are All Survivors.' " *Science*, Vol. 171, No. 3971 (Feb. 12, 1971), pp. 556–557. Copyright 1971 by the AAAS.

Science and Public Affairs (Bulletin of the Atomic Scientists)
Lewis, Richard S., "The Radioactive Salt Mine." *Science and Public Affairs* (Bulletin of the Atomic Scientists), Vol. 27, No. 6 (June 1971), pp. 27–30.

Science Service, Inc.
The following are reprinted with permission from *Science News*, the weekly news magazine of science and the applications of science:
Chamblin, Jay, "Rumblings from the Deep." *Science News*, Sept. 13, 1969. Copyright 1969 by Science Service, Inc.
Culliton, Barbara, "Noise-Polluting the Environment." *Science News*, Jan. 31, 1970. Copyright 1970 by Science Service, Inc.
Gross, Edward, "Digging Out from Under." *Science News*, Sept. 27, 1969. Copyright 1969 by Science Service, Inc.
"Northwest Passage." *Science News*, Sept. 27, 1969. Copyright 1969 by Science Service, Inc.

Stackpole Books
Still, Henry, *In Quest of Quiet.* Harrisburg, Pa.: Stackpole, 1970, pp. 9, 25, 27, 48, 53, 54, 62, 63, 70, 133, 152.

State University of New York
Wurster, Charles, "DDT: Danger to the Environment." *University Review*, Summer 1969, pp. 20–25.

Time, Inc.
The following are reprinted with permission from *Time*, The Weekly News-magazine:
"Fighting to Save the Earth from Man." *Time*, Feb. 2, 1970. Copyright Time Inc. 1970.
"The Peaceful Atom." *Time*, Jan. 19, 1970. Copyright Time Inc. 1970.
"The Black Tide." *Time*, Dec. 26, 1969. Copyright Time Inc. 1969.
"Menace in the Skies." *Time*, Jan. 27, 1967. Copyright Time Inc. 1967.
The following are reprinted from *Life* Magazine; © 1970 Time Inc.:
"The Dirty Dilemma of Oil Spills." *Life*, March 6, 1970.

Whipple, A. B. C., "An Ugly New Footprint in the Sand." *Life*, March 20, 1970.

University of Washington Press
Maxwell, Clyde, and Baker, C. M. Ann, *Molecular Biology and the Origin of Species*. Seattle: University of Washington Press, 1970.

University of Wisconsin Press
Rudd, Robert L., *Pesticides and the Living Landscape*. Madison: University of Wisconsin Press, 1964.

The Wall Street Journal
Benedict, Roger W., " 'Little Black Box': Fuel Cell, Long Seen as Electricity Source, Moves Ahead in Test." *The Wall Street Journal,* May 19, 1971, p. 1.

Franklin Watts, Inc.
Perry, John, *Our Polluted World—Call Man Survive?* New York: Franklin Watts, 1967.

REFERENCES

Abelson, Philip H. "Excessive Emotion about Detergents" (editorial), *Science*, Vol. 169, No. 3950 (September 11, 1970), p. 1033.

———. "Marine Pollution," *Science*, Vol. 171, No. 3966 (January 8, 1971), p. 21.

Albright, Edwin C., and Robert W. Allday, "Thyroid Carcinoma After Radiation Therapy for Adolescent Acne Vulgaris," *Journal of the American Medical Association* (hereafter *JAMA*), Vol. 199, No. 4 (January 23, 1967), pp. 280–81.

Altman, Lawrence K. "Japanese Diagnose Cadmium Disease," *The New York Times* (November 22, 1970), p. 73.

"Another SST," *Environment*, Vol. 13, No. 6 (July/August 1971), pp. 25–28.

A Primer on Waste Water Treatment, Federal Water Pollution Control Administration, U.S. Department of the Interior. Washington, D.C., 1969. Publication No. 1969 0–335–309.

Baron, Robert Alex. "Let Quiet Be Public Policy," *Saturday Review* (November 7, 1970), pp. 66–67.

Bazell, Robert J. "Lead Poisoning: Zoo Animals May Be the First Victims," *Science*, Vol. 173, No. 3992 (July 9, 1971), pp. 130–31.

Benarde, Melvin A. *Our Precarious Habitat*. New York: Norton, 1970.

Benedict, Roger W. " 'Little Black Box': Fuel Cell, Long Seen as Electricity Source, Moves Ahead in Tests," *The Wall Street Journal* (May 19, 1971), pp. 1, 14.

Berland, Theodore. *The Fight for Quiet*. Englewood Cliffs, N.J.: Prentice-Hall, 1970.

Binder, David. "Source of Fish Poisoning in Rhine Identified as Insecticide," *The New York Times* (June 26, 1969), p. 6.

Bird, David. "Rise in Dirt Particles Found in City's Air," *The New York Times* (September 20, 1971), p. 51.

Can Man Survive. Official Publication of the Centennial 1869–1969, The American Museum of Natural History. New York, 1969.

Carr, Donald E. *Death of the Sweet Waters*. New York: Norton, 1966.

Carter, Luther J. "The Global Environment: M.I.T. Study Looks for Danger Signs," *Science*, Vol. 169, No. 3946 (August 14, 1970), pp. 660–62.

Chamblin, Jay. "Rumblings from the Deep," *Science News*, Vol. 96, No. 11 (September 13, 1969).

Chase, Grafton D., and Arthur Abelson., (editorial), *Science*, Vol. 128, No. 3327 (October 3, 1958), p. 788.

Chow, Tsaihwa J., and John L. Earl. "Trend of Increasing Lead Aerosols in the Atmosphere," *Symposium on Geochemistry of Atmospheric Constituents* (annual meeting of the American Chemical Society, Houston, Texas, February 25, 1970).

Conard, Robert A., and Arobati Hicking. Abstract of "Medical Findings in Marshallese People Exposed to Fallout Radiation," *JAMA*, Vol. 192, No. 6 (May 10, 1965), p. 457.

"Control of Noises," *JAMA* (September 14, 1895); reprinted in *JAMA*, Vol. 213, No. 11 (September 14, 1970), p. 1771.

"Costing the Cacophony," *New Scientist*, Vol. 46, No. 700 (May 7, 1970), p. 269.

Craig, Roy. "Cloud on the Desert," *Environment*, Vol. 13, No. 6 (July/August 1971), pp. 20–24, 29–35.

Culliton, Barbara J. "Noise: Polluting the Environment," *Science News*, Vol. 97, No. 5 (January 31, 1970).

Curtis, Richard, and Elizabeth Hogan. *Perils of the Peaceful Atom*. New York: Doubleday, 1969.

Dillon, Jack. "Researchers Wrestle Challenge of City Noise," *The Christian Science Monitor* (September 13, 1965), p. 13.

"Downwind From the SST" (editorial), *The New York Times* (December 2, 1970), p. 46.

"Earth Watch," *Saturday Review* (November 7, 1970), p. 70.

Eisenbud, Merril. "Environmental Protection in the City of New York," *Science*, Vol. 170, No. 3959 (November 13, 1970), pp. 706–12.

Environmental Defense Fund advertisement, *The New York Times* (March 29, 1970), The Week in Review section, p. 6.

Environmental Health Problems. U.S. Public Health Service, U.S. Department of Health, Education, and Welfare. Washington, D.C., 1970. Publication No. 0–380–961.

"Environmental Quality: Its Significance in Our Environment" (editorial), *JAMA*, Vol. 214, No. 9 (November 30, 1970), p. 1717.

Esposito, John C. *Vanishing Air*. New York: Grossman, 1970. [The Ralph Nader Study Group Report on Air Pollution.]

Faust, Joan Lee. ". . . But Air Pollution Threatens," *The New York Times* (October 25, 1970), Arts and Leisure section, pp. 39, 40.

"Fighting to Save the Earth from Man," *Time* (February 2, 1970), pp. 56–63.

Fisher, Arthur. "Science Newsfront," *Popular Science* (October 1971), p. 46.

"French Condemn Insecticides," *The New York Times* (June 28, 1969), p. 6.

Fuller, Louis J. "Concluding Remarks," *Proceedings: The Third National Conference on Air Pollution* (hereafter *Proceedings*). Office of Legislative and Public Affairs National Center for Air Pollution Control. (Conference held on December 12–14, 1966.) Public Health Service Publication, pp. 458–59.

Gellen, Martin. "The Making of a Pollution-Industrial Complex," *Ramparts*, Vol. 8, No. 11 (May 1970), pp. 22–27. [Reprinted in Editors of Ramparts, *Eco-Catastrophe*. New York: Harper and Row, 1970. pp. 73–83.]

Gitlin, David. Letter, *The New York Times* (November 15, 1970) The Week in Review, p. 10.

Griffin, Joe L. Letter, *Science*, Vol. 172, No. 3982 (April 30, 1971), pp. 425–26.

Gross, Edward. "Digging Out from Under," *Science News*, Vol. 96, No. 13 (September 27, 1969).

Hammond, Allen L. "Mercury in the Environment," *Science*, Vol. 171, No. 3973 (February 26, 1971), pp. 788–89.

Harris, A. L. Letter, *New Scientist*, Vol. 46, No. 700 (May 7, 1970). p. 300–301.

Headley, J. C., and J. N. Lewis. *The Pesticide Problem: An Economic Approach to Public Policy.* Washington, D.C.: Resources for the Future, 1967.

Hechler, Ken. "TVA Ravages the Land," *National Parks and Conservation Magazine*, Vol. 45, No. 7 (July 1971), pp. 15–16.

Hill, Gladwin. "Purification of Nation's Waters Expected to be Long and Costly," *The New York Times* (March 17, 1970), pp. 1, 29.

_____. "Statistics Can Becloud the Pollution Picture," *The New York Times* (December 28, 1970), p. 26.

_____. "Texas Pollution Spurs Action by U.S.," *The New York Times* (January 19, 1970), p. 33.

Hofmann, Paul. "After a Century as Italy's Capital, the Eternal City Suffers Modern Agonies," *The New York Times* (September 21, 1970), p. 20.

Holden, Constance. "Nader Group Sees 'Water Wasteland'," *Science*, Vol. 172, No. 3982 (April 30, 1971), p. 455.

"Irradiation in Utero" (editorial), *JAMA*, Vol. 192, No. 5 (May 3, 1965), p. 410.

Jay, Anthony, and David Frost. *The English.* New York: Stein & Day, 1968).

Johnson, President Lyndon B. *Message to the Congress* (January 30, 1967).

Kenahan, Charles B. "Solid Waste—Resources out of Place," *Environmental Science and Technology*, Vol. 5, No. 7 (July 1971), pp. 594–600.

Kenworthy, E. W. "The Airlines Accept Pollution Deadline," *The New York Times* (January 21, 1970), pp. 1, 26.

Knapp, Carol E. "Recycling Sewage Biologically," *Environmental Science and Technology*, Vol. 5, No. 2 (February 1971), pp. 112–13.

Kurker, Charles. "Reducing Emissions from Refuse Disposal," *Journal of the Air Pollution Control Association*, Vol. 19, No. 2 (February 1969), pp. 69–72.

Landsberg, Helmut E. "Man-made Climatic Changes," *Science*, Vol. 170, No. 3964 (December 18, 1970), pp. 1265–74.

Larsen, Ralph I. "Relating Air Pollution Effects to Concentration and Control," *Journal of the Air Pollution Control Association*, Vol. 20, No. 4 (April 1970), pp. 214–25.

Lave, Lester B., and Eugene P. Seskin. "Air Pollution and Human Health," *Science*, Vol. 169, No. 3947 (August 21, 1970), pp. 723–33.

"Lead is Studied in Coastal Fish," *The New York Times* (December 27, 1970), p. 23.

Lear, John. "Teaching in the Big School," *Saturday Review* (January 2, 1971), pp. 63–66.

Leighton, Philip A. "Man and Air in California," printed in the Proceedings of the Statewide Conference on Man in California, 1980's by the University of California Extension Service, Berkeley, California, 1964.

Lewis, Howard R. *With Every Breath You Take.* New York: Crown, 1965.

Lewis, Richard S. "The Radioactive Salt Mine," *Science and Public Affairs* (Bulletin of the Atomic Scientists), Vol. XXVII, No. 6 (June 1971), pp. 27–30.

Lisco, Hermann, and Robert A. Conard. Abstract of "Chromosome Studies on Marshall Islanders Exposed to Fallout Radiation," *Science*, Vol. 157, No. 3787 (July 28, 1967), p. 445.

"London Curbs Fog," *Parade* (March 22, 1970), p. 9.

Lyons, Richard D. "Return to Detergents With Phosphates Urged by Government in Shift of Policy," *The New York Times* (September 16, 1971), pp. 1, 37.

McCaull, Julian. "Building a Shorter Life," *Environment*, Vol. 13, No. 7 (September 1971), pp. 2–15, 38–41.

Macdonald, Ross, and Robert Easton. "Santa Barbarans Cite An 11th Commandment: 'Thou Shalt Not Abuse the Earth'." *The New York Times Magazine* (October 12, 1969), pp. 32–33, 142–48, 151, 156.

Mallin, H. Martin, Jr. "Utility Concept of Solid Waste Handling makes

214

Gains," *Environmental Science and Technology*, Vol. 5, No. 9 (September 1971), pp. 752–53.

Marx, Leo. "American Institutions and Ecological Ideals," *Science*, Vol. 170, No. 3961 (November 27, 1970), pp. 945–52.

Maxwell, Clyde, and C. M. Ann Baker. *Molecular Biology and the Origin of Species.* Seattle, Wash.: University of Washington Press, 1970.

"Menace in the Skies," *Time* (January 27, 1967), pp. 48–52.

"Mercury in the Environment," *New Scientist*, Vol 47, No. 711 (July 23, 1970), p. 172.

Miller, Stanton S. "A Solid Waste Recovery System for all Municipalities," *Environmental Science and Technology*, Vol. 5, No. 2 (February 1971), pp. 109–11.

Mills, Clarence A. *Air Pollution and Community Health.* Boston: Christopher, 1954.

Montagu, Ashley. *The American Way of Life.* New York: Putnam's, 1967.

Montagu, Ashley, and Samuel S. Snyder. *Man and The Computer.* Philadelphia, Pa.: Auerbach, 1972.

Moore, Norman. "Pesticides Know no Frontiers," *New Scientist*, Vol. 46, No. 697 (April 16, 1970), pp. 114–15.

Moore, William W. "Reduction in Ambient Air Concentration of Fly Ash —Present and Future Prospects," *Proceedings*, pp. 170–78.

Morgan, George B., Guntis Ozolins and Elbert C. Tabor. "Air Pollution Surveillance Systems," *Science*, Vol. 170, No. 3955 (October 16, 1970), pp. 289–96.

Murozumi, M., Tsaihwa J. Chow and C. Patterson. "Chemical Concentrations of Pollutant Lead Aerosols, Terrestrial Dusts and Sea Salts in the Greenland and Antarctic Snow Strata," *Geochimica et Cosmochimica Acta*, Vol. 33 (1969), pp. 1247–94.

National Tuberculosis and Respiratory Disease Association. *Air Pollution Primer.* New York: The National Tuberculosis Association, 1969.

Needed: Clean Air. U.S. Department of Health, Education, and Welfare. Washington, D.C., 1969. Publication No. 138–E–69.

Nelson, Bryce. "Hiroshima after 25 Years: 'We Are All Survivors'," *Science*, Vol. 171, No. 3971 (February 12, 1971), pp. 556–57.

Nelson, Gaylord. "A Congressional View of the Problem," *Proceedings*, pp. 450–53.

Nelson, Gaylord A. "Our Polluted Planet," *The Progressive*, Vol. 33, No. 11 (November 1969), pp. 13–17.

Nisbet, Ian C. T., and Dallas Miner. "DDT Substitute," *Environment*, Vol. 13, No. 6 (July/August 1971), pp. 10–17.

"Northwest Passage," *Science News*, Vol. 96, No. 13 (September 27, 1969).

Novick, Sheldon. *The Careless Atom.* Boston: Houghton Mifflin, 1969.

Ottinger, Betty Ann. *What Every Woman Should Know—and Do—About Pollution: A Guide to Good Global Housekeeping.* Washington, D.C.: EP Press, 1970.

Pace, Eric. "Dutch Scientists Blame Polluted Dredged-Up Mud for Widespread Deaths of Seabirds 100 Miles Away," *The New York Times* (February 22, 1970), p. 4.

Perry, John. *Our Polluted World: Can Man Survive.* New York: Franklin Watts, 1967.

"Questions and Answers about Phosphates in Detergents and their Possible Effect on our Lakes and Streams." Proctor & Gamble Company advertisement, *Boston Evening Globe* (March 30, 1970), p. 7.

"Radiation and Radar Exposure Implicated in Down's Syndrome," *JAMA,* Vol. 194 (November 1, 1965), p. 34.

Rapoport, Roger. "Catch 24,400 (or, Plutonium Is My Favorite Element)," *Ramparts,* Vol. 8, No. 11 (May 1970), pp. 16–21. [Reprinted in Editors of Ramparts, *Eco-Catastrophe,* pp. 54–66.]

Rensberger, Boyce. "Mercury and Man: A Puzzle for Ecologists," *The New York Times* (May 21, 1971), p. 30.

Reston, Richard. "British Experts Warn Pollution Perils Life," *Los Angeles Times* (February 24, 1971), p. 26.

Rienow, Robert, and Leona Train Rienow. *Moment in the Sun: A Report on the Deteriorating Quality of the American Environment.* New York: Dial, 1967.

Ripley, Anthony. "Infants and Radioactive Sands: Small-Town Doctor Wins Fight," *The New York Times* (October 3, 1971), p. 75.

———. "Radioactive Building Sand Stirs Dispute," *The New York Times* (September 27, 1971), pp. 1, 15.

———. "Radioactive Sands Linked to Higher Death Rates," *The New York Times* (October 28, 1971), p. 27.

Robinson, E. W. *The Use of Radium in Consumer Products.* Washington, D.C.: Government Printing Office, 1968.

Rosenthal, David S., and Steven C. Beering. "Hypogonadism After Microwave Radiation," *JAMA,* Vol. 205, No. 4 (July 22, 1968), pp. 245–48.

Rudd, Robert L. *Pesticides and the Living Landscape.* Madison, Wis.: University of Wisconsin Press, 1964.

Ryan, William F. "A Congressional View of the Problem," *Proceedings,* pp. 342–47.

Schmeck, Harold M., Jr. "Caution on X-Ray: 'Don't Overdo It'," *The New York Times* (October 15, 1967), The Week in Review section, p. 6.

_____. "Scientist Links Mediocrity to Fetuses Damaged in Lax X-Ray Examinations," *The New York Times* (October 12, 1967), p. 35.

Seaborg, Glenn. "Do We Need Nuclear Power?" *The New York Times* (December 28, 1970), p. 31.

Semple, Robert B. "Great Lakes Pact Signed in Ottawa by Nixon, Trudeau," *The New York Times* (April 16, 1972), pp. 1, 3.

Sheaffer, John R. "Reviving the Great Lakes," *Saturday Review* (November 7, 1970), pp. 62–65.

Simon, Norman, and John Harley. "Skin Reactions From Gold Jewelry Contaminated With Radon Deposit," *JAMA*, Vol. 200, No. 3 (April 17, 1967), pp. 254–55.

Showdown. Federal Water Pollution Control Administration, U.S. Department of the Interior. Washington, D.C., 1968. Publication No. 0–320–380.

Small, William E. *Third Pollution: The National Problem of Solid Waste Disposal.* New York: Praeger, 1971.

Smith, Maynard E. "Reduction of Ambient Air Concentrations of Pollutants by Dispersion from High Stacks," *Proceedings*, pp. 151–60.

"Sonic-Boom Threat," *The Christian Science Monitor* (July 17, 1971), p. 14.

"Spectrum," *Environment*, Vol. 13, No. 6 (July/August 1971), p. 28.

"Spectrum," *Environment*, Vol. 13, No. 7 (September 1971), pp. 26–28.

Sporn, Philip. "Discussion of Preceding Three Papers," *Proceedings*, pp. 143–47.

Staples, James M. "Lead Particles in Air Seen as Peril to Brain, Blood and Bones," *The* (Newark, N.J.) *Evening News* (April 29, 1971), p. 26.

Stewart, Alice, and G. W. Kneale. "Radiation Dose Effects in Relation to Obstetric X-Rays and Childhood Cancers," *The Lancet*, 1970 Vol II (June 6, 1970), p. 1185.

Stewart, George R. *Not as Rich as You Think.* Boston: Houghton Mifflin, 1967.

Still, Henry. *In Quest of Quiet.* Harrisburg, Pa.: Stackpole Books, 1970.

Stuart, Peter C. "Pollution: What You Can Do," *The Christian Science Monitor* (February 18, 1971), p. 9.

Sullivan, Walter. "Oil Called Peril to Food Supply in Sea," *The New York Times* (January 16, 1970), p. 18.

"Swiss Scientist Estimates Seas Will Die in 25 Years," *The New York Times* (October 26, 1971), p. 5.

"The Black Tide," *Time* (December 26, 1969).

The City College of the City University of New York, *Proceedings of the Three-State Conference on Air Resource Management* (May 1967).

"The Dirty Dilemma of Oil Spills," *Life*, Vol. 68, No. 8 (March 6, 1970), p. 29.

The Effects of Air Pollution. U.S. Public Health Service, U.S. Department of Health, Education, and Welfare. Washington, D.C., 1968.

"The Hardin Follies" (editorial), *The New York Times* (July 24, 1970), p. 30.

The Menton Statement (signed by 2200 scientists from 23 countries, addressed to their "three and a half billion neighbors on planet earth," and handed to the U.N. secretary general on May 11, 1971).

"The Peaceful Atom," *Time* (January 19, 1970).

"The Price of Automobiles," *JAMA*, Vol. 214, No. 9 (November 30, 1970), p. 1717.

"The Ravaged Environment," *Newsweek* (January 26, 1970), pp. 30–45.

"The Role of Air Pollution in Chronic Obstructive Pulmonary Disease," *JAMA*, Vol. 214, No. 5 (November 2, 1970), pp. 894–99.

The Sources of Air Pollution and Their Control. U.S. Public Health Service, U.S. Department of Health, Education, and Welfare. (Washington, D.C., 1966). Publication No. 1548.

Toward a Quieter City. The Mayor's Task Force on Noise Control. New York, 1970.

"Trouble on Oily Waters" (editorial), *The New York Times* (July 19, 1970), p. 12.

Turner, Wallace. "California Plans Noise Regulation," *The New York Times* (Western Edition) (January 15, 1963), pp. 9, 11.

Udall, Stewart L. "Development of National Policy with Respect to Coal and Oil," *Proceedings,* pp. 128–30.

UNESCO Courier.

U.S. Senate Subcommittee on Air and Water Pollution, 1970.

Webster, Edward W. "Hazards of Diagnostic Radiology: A Physicist's Point of View," *Radiology,* Vol. 72, No. 4 (April 1959), p. 498.

Wegman, Leonard S. *A Proposal on Solid Waste Disposal.* The Business Council on Environment.

What You Can Do about Water Pollution. Federal Water Pollution Control Administration, U.S. Department of the Interior. Washington, D.C., 1967. Publication No. 0–265–805.

Whipple, A. B. C. "An Ugly New Footprint in the Sand," *Life*, Vol. 68, No. 10 (March 20, 1970), p. 20B.

Whiteside, Thomas. *Defoliation.* New York: Ballantine Books, 1970.

White-Stevens, Robert. Letter, *Science,* Vol. 170, No. 3961 (November 27, 1970), p. 928.

"Whitewash for Phosphates" (editorial), *The New York Times* (September 22, 1971), p. 46.

Wilcke, Gerd. "Detergent Companies Hail U.S. Step on Phosphates," *The New York Times* (September 16, 1971), p. 37.

Winn, Ira J. "Greetings from Los Angeles," *Natural History*, Vol. LXXX, No. 8 (October 1971).

Wurster, Charles. "DDT: Danger to the Environment," *University Review* (Summer 1969). Publication of the State University of New York.

"X Rays and Childhood Cancer" (editorial), *The Lancet*, 1968 Vol. I (March 16, 1968), pp. 577–78.

Zaret, Milton M. Letter, *JAMA*, Vol. 217, No. 4 (July 26, 1971), pp. 481–82.

Zinn, Walter H., Frank K. Pittman and John F. Hogerton. *Nuclear Power, U.S.A.* New York, 1964.